COMMUNITY CARE SITE SECURITY

Healthcare Security Field Manual

HSFM 2-1.0

David Corbin

Copyright © 2024 by David Corbin. All rights reserved.

Published by David P. Corbin. Salem, Massachusetts

Website: www.DavidPCorbin.com

No part of this publication may be reproduced, stored in a retrieval system, or transmitted in any form or by any means, electronic, mechanical, photocopying, recording, scanning, or otherwise, except as permitted under Section 107 or 108 of the 1976 United States Copyright Act, without the prior written permission of the author.

The material in this book is for informational purposes only. The advice and strategies contained herein may not be suitable for your situation. You should consult with a professional where appropriate. While the author has used his best efforts in preparing the material in this book, he makes no representations or warranties with respect to its accuracy or completeness, and specifically disclaims any implied warranties of merchantability or fitness for a particular purpose. No warranty may be created or extended by sales representatives or written sales materials. Neither the author nor publisher shall be liable for any loss of profit or any other damages, including but not limited to special, incidental, consequential, or other damages.

Company and product names mentioned herein are the trademarks or registered trademarks of their respective owners.

I dedicate this field manual to Constance (Connie) Packard, CHPA.
Friend, mentor, and kind soul.
May she rest in eternal peace.

ACKNOWLEDGEMENTS

A very special thank you to my wonderful beta readers from
the US, Canada, and the UK, respectively.

Michael Dunning, CEM, MEM, CHPA
Martin Green, CHPA
Laura Smith

Also, thank you to my LinkedIn friends who helped me figure out the final title for this manual.

Peta Mercieca, COHSProf
Mark Reed
Laura Smith (again)

PREFACE

I wrote this field manual to address the complex, challenging issue of providing security for community care sites. This is an issue that many of my colleagues and clients struggle with regularly. To make things even more interesting, they typically don't have the resources, human or financial, to implement a comprehensive security strategy.

If you're in the healthcare world, you know that community care sites, such as physician's offices, urgent care clinics, and even outpatient surgical centers are popping up faster than most organizations can keep up. I often have clients with over a hundred community care sites spread out over a wide geographic area. These clients regularly struggle to figure out how to provide a reasonable level of security for their sites with minimal resources.

Of course, each site comes with its own challenges, risks, and concerns raised by staff. It's a dilemma many healthcare organizations struggle with—from the independent physician's office to the enterprise with hundreds of sites. I also initially struggled with community care site security as a security director when I transitioned from a community hospital setting to a large urban hospital with over a hundred sites.

Through my work as both a consultant and a practitioner, I have developed an in-depth understanding of how community care sites operate. I have learned what worries community care site staff from interviewing hundreds of them across the US. Further, through my research, I have a better understanding of the security and resource issues that international community care sites face. I have also uncovered, through research, trial, and error, from clients and colleagues how to create effective and sustainable community care site security.

The intent behind this field manual is to provide clear, concise guidance to anyone, from a practice manager to an enterprise security leader, to improve community care site security. I want my readers to be able to pick up this manual and gain insights, strategies, and tactics that they can immediately apply in their own organization.

Lastly, because many readers of my previous publication, the *Patient Violence Prevention and Mitigation Field Manual*, are from outside the US in Canada, England, Australia, Singapore, and beyond, this manual is written with a broad, international audience in mind.

CONTENTS

Acknowledgements v
Preface vii
Introduction xiii

Chapter 1 The Community Care Site Operational Environment 1

    1.1   Overview 1
    1.2   Operational Variables 2

Chapter 2 Physical Security Strategy 6

    2.1   Overview 6
    2.2   Strategy 6
    2.3   Consistency 6
    2.4   Layered Approach 7

Chapter 3 Exterior Physical Security Measures 9

    3.1   Overview 9
    3.2   Lighting 9
    3.2.1 Overview 9
    3.2.2 Definitions 9
    3.2.3 Standards & Recommended Lighting Levels 10
    3.2.4 Lighting Assessment 12
    3.2.5 Next Steps 15
    3.3   Bollards – Protecting Against Vehicle Impact 15
    3.3.1 Overview 15
    3.3.2 Bollard Selection and Standards 16
    3.4   Maintenance 17
    3.5   Exterior Access Control 17
    3.5.1 Overview 17
    3.5.2 Fencing 17
    3.5.3 Fencing Considerations 18

	3.5.4	Doors, Roof Hatches, and Windows 19
	3.6	Electronic Security 21
	3.6.1	Overview 21
	3.7	Security Cameras 22
	3.7.1	Overview 22
	3.7.2	Camera Placement 22
	3.7.3	Camera Selection 22
	3.7.4	Video Recording 23
	3.7.5	Video Monitoring 23
	3.8	Card Access System 24
	3.8.1	Lockdown Capabilities 25

Chapter 4 Interior Physical Security Measures 26

	4.1	Overview 26
	4.2	Check-In/Waiting Area 26
	4.3	Treatment Area 28
	4.4	Emergency Shelter Room(s) 29
	4.5	Building Alarm System 30
	4.5.1	Additional Components 31
	4.5.2	System Codes and Response 32

Chapter 5 Site Operational Security 33

	5.1	Overview 33
	5.2	Opening and Closing Procedures 33
	5.3	Cleaning Service 33
	5.4	Pre-Appointment Communications 34
	5.5	Wait Times 34
	5.6	Diversions 34
	5.7	Code word 34
	5.8	See Something, Say Something 35
	5.9	Conclusion 35

Chapter 6 Emergency Preparedness 36

	6.1	Overview 36
	6.2	Emergency Notification Method 36
	6.3	Essential Security-Related Emergency Plans 37
	6.3.1	Active Shooter/Active Threat 37
	6.3.2	External Threat 38

  6.3.3 Violent Person 38
  6.3.4 Conclusion 39

Chapter 7 *Workplace Violence in the Community Care Setting* 40

  7.1 Types of Violence in the Community Care Setting 40
  7.1.1 Common Types of Violence in the Community Care Setting 40
  7.1.2 Less Common Types of Violence in the Community Care Setting 41
  7.1.3 Rare Types of Violence in the Community Care Setting 42
  7.2 Violence Prevention & Mitigation in the Community Care Setting 43
  7.2.1 Violence Risk Assessment 43
  7.2.2 Violence Risk Assessment Analysis 45
  7.2.3 Violence Risk Assessment – External Consultants 46
  7.3 Essential Violence Prevention & Mitigation Measures 46
  7.3.1 Overview 46
  7.3.2 Encourage Reporting 46
  7.3.3 Investigate Incidents and Support Victims of Violence 46
  7.3.4 Support Employee Wellbeing 47
  7.3.5 Provide De-escalation Training 47
  7.3.6 Plan in Advance for Concerning Patients 48
  7.3.7 Mitigate Firearms Risks 49

Chapter 8 *Community Care Site Security Operations Models* 51

  8.1 Overview 51
  8.2 Improved Security Operations Models 52
  8.2.1 Improved Practice and Risk/Operations Manager - Led Security Operations ... 52
  8.2.2 Improved Enterprise-Led Security Operations 54
  8.2.3 Conclusion 57

Chapter 9 *Practice/Operations/Risk Manager-Led Security Operations* 58

  9.1 Overview 58
  9.2 Security Services 58
  9.3 Liaison with Law Enforcement 60
  9.4 Practice Manager Daily Security Operations 61
  9.4.1 Practice Manager Monthly/Quarterly/Annual Operations 62
  9.5 Operations/Risk Manager-Led Security Operations 62
  9.5.1 Delegation of Security Operations 62
  9.5.2 Weekly Security Operations 62
  9.5.3 Monthly/Quarterly/Annual Operations 64

Chapter 10 Enterprise Security Operations 65

    10.1   Overview 65
    10.2   Community Care Security Team Strategy 65
    10.2.1 Community Oriented Policing Approach 66
    10.2.2 Community-Oriented Policing Effectiveness 66
    10.2.3 Adapting Community-Oriented Policing for Community Care Security 67

Chapter 11 Establishing the Community Care Security Team 69

    11.1   Leadership 69
    11.2   Staffing 69

Chapter 12 The Community Care Security Officer (CCSO) 71

    12.1   Overview 71
    12.2   Selection 71
    12.3   Training 72
    12.4   CCSO Operations 72
    12.4.1 Field-Based Team 72
    12.4.2 Daily Operations 72
    12.4.3 Monthly/Quarterly/Annual Operations 74
    12.4.4 Special Operations - Security Details 74
    12.5   Essential CCSO Equipment 75
    12.5.1 Field Communications 75

Chapter 13 Community Care Site Intelligence Operations 76

    13.1   Overview 76
    13.2   Intelligence Collection Technology 76
    13.3   Intelligence Alerting 77
    13.4   Field Intelligence 77

Final Thoughts 79
About The Author 81
References 83

INTRODUCTION

Community care sites are an important part of the overall delivery of healthcare to millions of people every day. But what are community care sites? For the purposes of this manual, community care sites are physical locations, separate from a hospital, where non-acute healthcare is delivered close to where patients live. Examples of such sites include, but are not limited to: doctor's offices, physical therapy practices, urgent care clinics, and outpatient surgical suites. These sites may be small offices, large multi-level buildings, or campuses.

This manual is designed to help improve the security of community care sites- from physical security to workplace violence prevention and emergency preparedness for security events. I designed this manual to be read and understood by anyone responsible for community care site security- from a practice manager to an enterprise healthcare leader. This approach aligns with the spirit of the US Army field manuals that serve as the inspiration for this manual. In true field manual fashion, the information, insights, and guidance I present here are clear, concise, and actionable.

I suggest that non-security community care leadership read Chapters 1 through 9 to build a solid understanding of everything ranging from workplace violence risk factors to leading their organization's security operations. Security leaders, however, should read the entire manual to gain a comprehensive understanding of how to build and lead security operations in collaboration with site leadership.

After reading this manual, I recommend that you and your respective team(s) conduct assessments of each site using the guidance outlined in chapters 2-7. This process will assist you in identifying a range of issues, from poor lighting to missing policies and procedures. Also, don't forget to calculate the violence safety gap for each site as outlined in Chapter 1 under the "Time" operational variable.

Next, the assessments can be used to map out and prioritize improvements for one site or across a large enterprise-level organization with hundreds of sites. In many cases, the improvements, whether related to training or physical security, will need to be phased in over time. The key is to make a plan, identify key milestones, and maintain momentum until improvements are completed.

In terms of evaluating your community care site security operations, a similar process can be used as outlined above. If you're a community care leader, read chapter 9. If you're a security leader, read chapters 9-13. This operational assessment should also result in the identification of improvements needed and a phased plan for implementing improvements.

The goal of this manual is to educate and empower you to improve the security of your community care sites for the safety and wellbeing of your staff and patients. I also want this manual to serve as a reference that you can pull off the shelf anytime you need further guidance, ideas, or inspiration.

CHAPTER 1

The Community Care Site Operational Environment

1.1 Overview

Community care sites are being established at an ever-increasing pace within the United States and beyond. This expansion is due to both cost-effectiveness for healthcare organizations and preferences of the patients they serve (Michas, 2022).

The types of community care sites vary, but they generally include general medical practices/doctor's offices, community care surgical sites, urgent care, and specialty care clinics (e.g., physical therapy and dialysis). In the US and in Canada, these care sites are operated by hospitals, healthcare organizations, physician's organizations, individuals, retailers, and others. In the UK, community care clinics are primarily operated by the National Health Service (NHS) followed by private healthcare companies and non-profit organizations.

As of 2022, there were a total of 643,000 community care sites in the United States and 209,661 in Canada (Michas, 2022, 2023). Updated community care site statistics were not readily available for the UK at the time of this publication. In the US, community care sites employ 7.4 million staff and account for $1 trillion in annual revenue (Michas, 2022). Globally, the community care services market is expected to grow from $3.32 billion in 2022 to $5.33 billion in 2027, according to the Community Care Services Global Market Report 2023.

Further, retailers are increasingly entering the community care healthcare market, establishing both freestanding clinics and care sites within existing stores. As of March 2023, there were 1,801 retail clinics within 44 states in the US, with most clinics in the Southeast and Midwest (Definitive Healthcare, 2023). Most of these clinics are owned by large retailers such as CVS, Kroger, Walgreens and Walmart (*Retail clinics target chronic diseases: AHA*).

Apart from larger sites, most community care locations don't have on-site security staff. When staff at these sites need assistance with a security-related emergency, they call the local police. Further, many of these sites lack basic security elements, such as staff de-escalation training, security emergency procedures, duress/panic alarms, and building alarm systems. Even when community care sites are connected to a hospital or healthcare system, the sheer number and wide geographic distribution of these sites is often too much for the organization's security department to support.

The community care site model is an approach to healthcare delivery that shows no signs of slowing down anytime soon. Therefore, it is critical that healthcare leaders responsible for security at these sites understand the operational variables that can influence risk exposure for staff, patients, and site assets.

As you work through this chapter, you should take the time to write down how each of these variables applies to sites within your organization. Think about how each variable might support or impede your efforts to enhance the security posture of your sites. These notes will ultimately be helpful in determining where to focus your efforts when building out your community care security program.

1.2 Operational Variables

Below is a list of common variables impacting community care site security and, therefore, your efforts to enhance and/or establish a community care site security program.

A. **Time:** Time is one of the most critical factors in planning community care site security measures. The absence of security staff at most sites creates a violence safety gap. The violence safety gap is the amount of time between a violent event beginning until police arrive. There's no fixed formula to calculate the violence safety gap, but here are three factors to consider when estimating this gap for each site:

- Police Response Time: A recent review of police priority one call response times in eight large US cities by data analyst Jeff Asher in 2023 found increases in all of them- some more dramatic than others- from 2019 to 2022. The factors that impact police response times to priority one emergencies in the US are also playing out globally and include low police staffing levels and increasing demand for routine and emergency services.
- Ability to Summon Police Quickly: The faster the police can be notified of an incident, the faster they can be dispatched to respond. Staff must know the emergency number to call, their address and their exact location within the building. Voice over IP (VoIP) phone systems must transmit accurate locations of emergency callers within the building to the emergency call center. Access to a panic alarm system, particularly a body-worn system that is monitored by an alarm monitoring center, can get police rolling quickly before staff can get to a phone, improving police response time.
- Training: Staff must understand how to communicate the nature of the emergency clearly so that police understand the incident severity. They must also know not

to wait until the situation is out of control to call the police. The earlier the police can be notified, the better. Further, staff who downplay the incident and/or who fail to state the incident is in progress can inadvertently slow police response.

The security measures employed at each site can help to shorten and/or bridge the violence safety gap. For example, if staff are equipped with body-worn panic/duress alarms, they can summon police assistance very quickly in an emergency, shortening the gap. Also, if there are strong physical security measures in place between the waiting area and treatment area, staff and patients can be kept safe from an out-of-control patient in the waiting area. Time should be a key consideration in any security strategies and tactics for community care sites.

B. **Security**: Most sites, hospitals, and/or healthcare enterprises don't have the resources to put security staff at each community care site. Further, security staff cannot effectively respond to emergencies at most sites given their varied geographic locations and the lack of emergency response vehicles.

Community care sites that are not affiliated with a hospital or healthcare organization may have no security team at all. It's not uncommon in the US to see an independent multi-site community care practice with no one directly responsible for security. Retail community care sites in large retail stores typically have security departments, usually referred to as loss prevention or asset protection, to lean on for security support.

Without on-site security or nearby security available to respond, community care sites rely heavily on local police to assist with routine and emergency security situations. The response time and support offered by each law enforcement agency can vary widely depending on their location, resources, and demands on those resources. It's critical to understand what can reasonably be expected from local law enforcement in terms of support and response when planning site security. Open lines of communication with local law enforcement leadership are key to this understanding.

C. **Political**: The political variable includes the distribution of power and responsibility within and outside your organization. It's key to understand the political landscape you are navigating if you want to be successful in your efforts to enhance or establish a community care security program. An example of an internal political variable is a power struggle between the hospital and a physician's group that operates several community care practices. If the physician's group wants the hospital's budget to pay for new security measures, your efforts may be doomed unless the hospital agrees. An external political variable may be a conflict between the security measures the hospital wants to implement at a clinic and property restrictions imposed by the building landlord. In the UK, historical Listed Building restrictions imposed by law can limit the ability to implement certain security measures.

D. **Community**: This variable can be viewed from both the internal and external community perspectives.

The internal community generally consists of staff working within the community care setting and the patients they serve. This community plays an important role in developing and shaping the security program. That's because staff buy-in is needed to establish an effective security program. Security measures won't work if staff override them, don't understand how to use them, or find that they don't fit with the site's operations. Patients served by the site also need to be considered in your security planning. You should understand how the presence of certain security measures might impact their feelings of comfort and trust.

The external community generally consists of the homes, businesses, local government, and people who are in the area surrounding your community care sites. Community care sites are designed to serve a wide range of patients and communities and are usually spread out across many locations. They may be in a low crime area, a high crime area, or anywhere in between. Security measures that work in a low crime area may not be appropriate for a high crime area. Security measures should be tailored to both the external and internal communities for these reasons. However, to tailor your security measures appropriately, you must first understand these communities.

E. **Economic:** This variable also has an internal and external component.

Internally, the overall finances of the organization and available funding for security resources can make or break your security program. That's why it's important to approach and plan your community care security program strategically. A risk-based, multi-year strategic security plan is more likely to get support from senior leadership than a piecemeal approach.

The external economic factors playing out within the communities that community care sites serve can directly impact security. Locations where much of the population lives in poverty are vulnerable, and have high unemployment rates may be more likely to have high crime rates, including property crime and violent crime. The stresses of such an environment will also follow patients into these sites, impacting staff and operations.

F. **Social:** The social variable describes societies in the external environment. A society is a population who live in a defined community, have a common culture, a sense of identity, and are under the same government. Social issues that can impact community care sites can occur at the local, regional, or national level. For example, a clinic providing what are considered controversial medical services to a portion of society may increase the security risks of that site. Understanding the social factors, both established and dynamic, within the communities where community care sites are located is a key part of developing security measures.

G. **Information:** Establishing and maintaining your community care security program requires leveraging both internal and external information.

<u>Internal information</u> should always involve two-way communications. Security and/or site leadership must frequently communicate with staff to update them on new risks, procedures, or security measures. Site staff must also keep security and/or site leadership updated on any security issues or concerns and should file incident reports for security events as needed.

<u>External communications</u> must also be two-way. Security and/or site leadership should establish a good working relationship with local law enforcement to collect and share information critical to the security of each site.

H. **Physical Environment:** The physical environment of community care sites can vary widely. Community care sites may be housed in their own large freestanding multistory building, as a tenant in an office park, in a storefront, etc. When a community care site is a tenant in a building, office park, or another location, there may be little control over exterior lighting issues, general building security, and other factors. Conversely, a large community care freestanding building may have its own parking structure and multiple clinics and services with different operating hours. Every site comes with its own challenges and security measures should be tailored to address each unique environment.

All these variables should be collected and carefully analyzed when building or enhancing your community care security program. A strategic approach to your program that factors in these variables will help you to avoid foreseeable pitfalls, set realistic expectations, effectively communicate risks, and garner necessary support.

Chapter 2

Physical Security Strategy

2.1 Overview

Physical security measures at community care sites are critical to keeping staff, patients, and others safe in the care environment. Further, physical security plays a key role in bridging the violence safety gap mentioned in Chapter 1. When layered physical security is done right, it can keep staff, patients, and others safe until help can arrive.

2.2 Strategy

There are two key elements of physical security strategy for community care sites: consistency and a layered approach to security measures. Consistency means that each community care site has a minimum baseline of security measures in place to keep staff safe. The layered approach to security measures means that one element of physical security is stacked upon the next. These layers of security, working together, create a stronger overall level of security than if each element was functioning alone.

2.3 Consistency

Consistency is key when planning physical security measures to protect more than one community care site. Oftentimes, organizations implement disparate measures across their care sites, resulting in different levels of security at sites facing the same level of risk. For example, a newly established care site may have a card access system, cameras, and panic alarms while the care site across town has a broken building alarm system and doors secured with mechanical push-button locks.

The minimum baseline of physical security measures should be based on the average overall security and violence risks facing the community care sites within the organization. Once this baseline is established, efforts must be made to get each care site to meet the baseline in a reasonable timeframe.

Next, additional physical security measures should be layered on top of this baseline when the risks to a site(s) is higher than average. For example, an organization may establish baseline security measures at each site consisting of a building alarm system, panic/duress buttons, and locked doors between the waiting area and treatment area. If a site within that organization is located within a high crime area and/or treats a high-risk patient population, additional security measures may be added, such as body-worn panic/duress alarms, reinforced clear barriers at the check-in desk, security cameras, and an exterior door lockdown button.

Consistency also simplifies planning new site security measures and can help reduce liability exposure that can stem from providing distinct levels of protection for staff and patients against the same level of risk.

2.4 Layered Approach

The layered approach to physical security is often compared to the layers of an onion. Each layer of the onion's skin and internal layers work together to protect the core of the onion. The core in this case is the staff, patients, and the assets of the site. The best way to describe how these layers work to provide security is using the 5 Ds method: Deter, Detect, Deny, Delay, Defend. Each of these elements is described in more depth below.

- **Deter:** The first line of defense is deterrence. Deterrence involves discouraging people who may pose a risk to the site and its occupants from attempting to enter the exterior or interior perimeter of the site. The idea here is to send a message to potential bad actors that the site is well-protected and that attempts to enter the perimeter will be difficult.
- **Detect:** The next line of defense is detection. The earlier a potential threat can be identified, the sooner it can be addressed by police, security, and/or additional physical security measures, like a lockdown of the perimeter. After hours, a building alarm system serves to detect when someone is breaking into the facility and contacts police through a central station. The threat of detection also serves as a deterrent to bad actors.
- **Deny:** Denial means preventing the threat from getting through a layer of the perimeter. Perimeter measures such as locked employee-only and emergency exit doors prevent a threat from getting into the treatment area of the site from the outside. Locked doors in the waiting area keep a bad actor from gaining unauthorized access to the treatment area.
- **Delay:** Delay means slowing down the threat once it has made it through a layer of the perimeter. For example, if a patient has entered the site through the unlocked main entrance and is demanding to see a doctor, the locked doors leading to the treatment area will slow him down in attempting to access the area. If the glass on the windows of those doors is laminated, it will slow his ability to smash the windows to unlock the door. The idea behind the delay is to buy time for the police or security to arrive and address the threat.

- **Defend:** Defend involves the police or the security team arriving to address and stop the threat. In some cases, addressing and stopping the threat may be initially handled by site staff who are trained in de-escalation and basic physical self-defense/restraint techniques.

When security measures are planned with the 5 Ds in mind using a layered approach, the effects of each layer are strengthened, resulting in greater protection for staff, patients, and assets. The sections that follow detail the security layers of the exterior and interior perimeter and how they can be leveraged to create a solid baseline of security and enhanced security for community care sites.

Chapter 3

Exterior Physical Security Measures

3.1 Overview

The exterior of a building or site generally consists of the parking areas and/or garage, landscaping, sidewalks, and the outside perimeter of the building. This is where layered security for a community care site begins. This chapter walks through the layered elements of exterior physical security, how to evaluate them, and how to enhance them.

3.2 Lighting

3.2.1 Overview

Proper exterior lighting at community care sites is an often-overlooked element of security. Good lighting creates feelings of safety among staff and patients and help deter criminal activity. Generally, lights should be bright enough to allow people to see clearly at night, should be evenly distributed with minimal dark spots, and operated by a photocell sensor. This section outlines simple ways to evaluate existing lighting conditions for various areas and how to improve them.

3.2.2 Definitions

These definitions are for purposes of clarifying terms used in this section:

Foot-Candle: The illuminance on a one square foot surface from a uniform source of light.

Kelvin: A measure of the color "temperature" of a light source. The higher the Kelvin rating (symbol "K"), the whiter the light. The scale for commercial lighting typically ranges from 2000K (warm white) to 6500K (daylight).

Lumen: A unit of luminous flux equal to the light emitted in a unit solid angle (a three-dimensional measure) by a uniform point source of one candle intensity.

Luminous flux: A measure of the power of visible light produced by a light source.

Lux: One lux is equal to one lumen per square meter.

Uniformity Ratio: The ratio between the average illumination in an area and the minimum or maximum illumination in each area.

3.2.3 Standards & Recommended Lighting Levels

The Illuminating Engineering Society (IES) is viewed as the authority in lighting standards. IES publishes a variety of lighting standards for various applications. Table 1 lists the recommended illumination levels for the areas noted along with their accompanying uniformity ratios according to the 2022 Illuminating Engineering Society publication, *Recommended Practice: Lighting Exterior Applications*.

Table 1

Location	Horizontal Illuminance Lower Limit- Upper Limit (foot-candles/lux)	Vertical Illuminance Lower Limit-Upper Limit (foot-candles)	Ratio (Avg:Min)
Building Entrances	3-5 / 32-54	1 – 3 / 11-32	5:1
Walking Surfaces- adjacent to exits/architecture	1-3 / 11-32	N/A	10:1
Stairs and ramps	4 – 5 / 43-54	N/A	5:1

The lighting recommendations for community care sites below are based on the IES standards, a recent IES publication, and general Crime Prevention Through Environmental Design (CPTED) best practices. These recommendations also consider the need to create the perception of enhanced safety and security for patients and staff while creating a perception of enhanced risk for bad actors.

1. Responsible Outdoor Lighting: Lighting improvements should follow the IES five principles for responsible outdoor lighting listed below (IES, 2022):

   a. Useful: All lighting should have a clear purpose.

   b. Targeted: Light should be directed only where it is needed. Avoid light trespass into areas where it is not necessary. Minimize glare and light directed upwards whenever possible.

   c. Low light levels: Light should be no brighter than necessary.

   d. Controlled: Lighting should only be used when it is useful.

   e. Color: Warmer color lighting should be used when possible.

2. Lighting Controls:

   a. All outdoor lighting, including at building entrances, should be controlled by photocell sensors and not by timers, which cannot effectively keep pace with gradual fluctuations in daylight hours across seasons.

   b. Motion sensors should be used on pole and building mounted fixtures where possible to align with IES responsible lighting principles. These sensors should dim lights to about 60% of full illumination when motion is not detected (IES, 2022). Motion sensor lights are also useful in security lighting as they can indicate to police the presence of a person or vehicle in the area after normal business hours.

3. Specific Areas: Community care sites should have sufficient lighting for both safety (i.e.- trip hazards, pedestrian/vehicle interactions) and security purposes.

   a. **Building entrances**

      i. Lighting at building entrances, including employee-only entry points, fire exits, and other non-public entry point should be at a minimum of 3 foot-candles/32 lux of horizontal illumination in the immediate area of the door (typically an overhead fixture) at a color temperature of 4000-K. The primary public entrance(s) should be illuminated to 4 foot-candles/43 lux or higher to make them stand out as primary entry points (IES, 2022).

b. **Walking surfaces:**

   i. Walking surfaces surrounding the building should generally be illuminated to a minimum of 1 foot-candle/11 lux at 4000-K color temperature at both the ground level and at the 3 foot/~1 meter height to provide adequate illumination of the surroundings, like landscaped areas and other pedestrians. Consider utilizing a combination of existing pole-mounted lights, bollard mounted lights, and building-mounted lighting fixtures to accomplish goal illumination levels (IES, 2022).

   ii. Stairs and ramps should be illuminated at a minimum of 4 foot-candles/43 lux at a 4000-K color temperature using focused, low-height LED fixtures directing light onto these surfaces (IES, 2022).

c. **Parking Areas**

   i. Parking areas, including both patient and employee parking lots, should generally be illuminated to a minimum of 1 foot-candle/11 lux at 4000-K color temperature and a maximum 5:1 uniformity ratio to provide adequate illumination of the pavement and surroundings, such as vehicles, pedestrians, and landscaping (IES, 2022). Goal lighting levels may be accomplished by utilizing a combination of existing pole mounted lights and building-mounted light fixtures.

   According to a 2019 study by the Illuminating Engineering Society, "an average pavement illuminance of 2 lux [.185 foot-candle] can ensure a higher visual performance and higher perceptions of safety, comfort, and visibility for all parking lot users (pedestrians and drivers)" (IES, 2019). The study also highlighted the importance of the lighting color temperature as measured on the Kelvin (K) temperature scale, in parking lots, finding that, "at an average pavement illuminance of 2 lux, the 5000-K and 3000-K LEDs enabled higher perceptions of safety, comfort, and visibility for all parking lot users" (IES, 2019).

3.2.4 Lighting Assessment

To conduct a basic assessment of the lighting levels at a given location, you don't need much more than an inexpensive illuminance meter, a pen, and a basic map. Outlined below are the steps to conduct this assessment:

1. **Light Measurement Tool:** To measure lighting levels, use an inexpensive illuminance meter purchased on Amazon that has a wide lux/footcandle range and an illuminated

display. While this type of light meter may not be a professional grade light meter used by a lighting engineer, it will give you an idea of the levels of illumination in the key exterior locations mentioned in this section. From this point, you can evaluate what areas need additional lighting.

2. **Mapping Light Fixtures:** Use a map of the areas being audited to mark the measurements recorded by your light meter. These marked measurements will also help you to determine the uniformity of lighting. You also want to mark the locations of exterior light fixtures, note the general mount type (i.e.- wall pack, pole mounted) and the type of light, if known (i.e.- high pressure sodium, LED). Light fixture types are outlined under #4 below. If you can't get a map from your facilities team, you can draw one yourself or use Google Maps to make one.

3. **Light Measurements:** To take light measurements, hold the light meter in front of you facing upwards in total darkness (typically 70-100 minutes after sunset) and move from one end of the area being surveyed to the other. Take measurements every 10-20 feet/3-6 meters and record them on your map or drawing.

   You can also take vertical measurements if you wish by holding the light at eye level and facing the sensor vertically. Vertical measurements are helpful for evaluating lighting at building entrances and parking lots. Vertical lighting helps people to see and identify faces and vehicles.

   If you're surveying a large area like a parking lot, move and take measurements in a grid pattern for uniformity. Don't worry about being perfect here- you're just trying to evaluate whether lighting is sufficient and, if it's not, where additional lighting is needed. Leave it to the professionals to determine how to address your findings.

4. **Fixture Evaluation:** Determine what types of light fixtures are in place around the facility. Make note during the audit of any light fixtures that are blocked or impeded by overgrowth of trees and shrubs. These fixtures are not effective if they cannot deliver lighting to the intended area. Ongoing proactive landscape maintenance is a critical part of ensuring lighting effectiveness. The typical fixture types are outlined below.

   a. Bollard or ground lighting: Mounted on low poles (approximately waist height) and are meant to illuminate the ground and/or walking surfaces.

   b. Flood light: Mounted to the building to illuminate a certain area of interest.

   c. Pole-mounted: Mounted to a light pole with the light directed downwards or towards a certain location (spotlight).

d. Wall pack: Usually mounted to the side of a building and are typically square with the light on the bottom half of the square.

5. **Lighting Type Identification:** Each fixture has a light source that can vary in output and clarity. Below is a quick guide to help identify what type of light source is being used. Ask facilities or maintenance leadership responsible for the site for the type(s) of lighting in place if it's unclear. Facilities leadership can also tell you whether the lights are on a timer or operated by photocell.

    a. High Pressure Sodium: Yellowish warm light range of 1900-2000K. Low efficiency, frequent maintenance, warmup period to full output.

    b. Low Pressure Sodium: Yellowish warm light around 1800K. Low efficiency, frequent maintenance, warmup period to full output.

    c. High Pressure Mercury: White light range of 3500-4500K. Low efficiency, frequent maintenance, warmup period to full output.

    d. LED (light emitting diode): White light range of 3100-6500K+. High efficiency, very infrequent maintenance, no warmup period to full output.

    e. Metal Halide fixtures: Wide range of 3000K-20,000K. Lower efficiency than LED, frequent maintenance, warm up period, high heat/UV output.

    Note that High-Pressure Sodium, High-Pressure Mercury, and Metal Halide lighting were phased out by 2017 by the European Union. The United States, Canada, and other countries have phased out, have plans to phase out, or are implementing efficiency standards on many non-LED lighting technologies.

    Most facilities with modern or upgraded lighting are moving to LED fixtures as they can render clear, white light using far less energy and with much less maintenance. LED fixtures also enhance performance of exterior security cameras, providing clearer images and accurate color rendering. In some areas, local utility company programs may incentivize or provide significant rebates to re-lamp exterior (and even interior) lighting.

6. **Lighting Uniformity Calculation:** Once the site audit is completed, the next step is to determine lighting uniformity. To do this, add up the measurements from a particular area, like the perimeter of the building or one parking lot and divide by the number of measurements you took to get the average illumination. Next, look at the minimum level of lighting in the area as a comparison point. For example, the area directly under a light

fixture might have measured at 3 foot-candles/32 lux and the area 20 feet/6 meters away may have measured at 1 foot candle/11 lux. The uniformity ratio in this case would be 3:1. Table 1 in this section is a helpful reference in determining whether the uniformity ratio is within minimum guidelines.

3.2.5 Next Steps

Once you've completed your lighting audit, you should meet with your leadership and facilities leadership to discuss your findings and recommendations for improvement. Again, a lighting engineer and/or trusted lighting vendor professional can help with addressing your findings.

Note that community care sites housed in leased buildings/spaces may encounter challenges with the building owner/management regarding inadequate lighting concerns. In these cases, educating them about lighting standards and presenting them with the lighting audit conducted at the site may be a good strategy.

3.3 Bollards – Protecting Against Vehicle Impact

3.3.1 Overview

Bollards are an essential element of exterior physical security for community care sites- especially since many of these sites are located within immediate or very close proximity to parking lots (such as a storefront urgent care clinic) and roadways.

Bollards can take many forms, but they are typically poles anchored in the ground that are designed to stop vehicles from driving into a building. This threat is more common than you may think. According to the Storefront Safety Council, there were over 100 storefront crashes daily in the United States in 2022. Of these crashes, 46% resulted in injuries and 8% resulted in fatalities (Crash Statistics: Storefront Safety Council, 2022). This is not to mention the damage to the building and the resulting operational impacts.

Bollards should be placed in exterior locations around a community care building or storefront where there is a risk of vehicle impact, such as the following:

- Along the sides of the building exposed to parking areas- regardless of whether there is a wall, window, or door exposed.
- Across portions of the building that are exposed to moving vehicle traffic within the parking lot, such as drop-off areas.
- Alongside building perimeter locations immediately exposed to adjacent street traffic, especially near intersections, where accidents can occur or where an intersecting road may point vehicles directly at the building.
- Where critical infrastructure on the perimeter of the building needs to be protected from nearby vehicle impacts, such as a natural gas main connection point.

3.3.2 Bollard Selection and Standards

Once you have established where bollards need to be installed, it's important to install the correct bollards for the level of risk. For example, bollards protecting your building from vehicles in a parking lot may require a lower speed protection rating than bollards protecting your building from vehicles in a nearby intersection.

Not all bollards are created equal and simply bolting a pole to the ground won't result in any real protection from vehicle impact. For those with an eye towards improved aesthetics, bollards come in all shapes, sizes, and features. There are also options to place crash-rated planters, benches, and other architectural and landscape features that can protect your building from vehicle impacts.

Consulting a qualified professional is advised when determining the right level of protection and ensuring bollard placement doesn't conflict with accessibility requirements. However, it's also important to understand the standards around bollard ratings, placement, spacing and protection. Here are some standards and guidance to familiarize yourself with:

- United States and Canada:
  - ASTM International:
    - F2656/F2656M-20: Standard Test Method for Crash Testing of Vehicle Security Barriers
    - F3016/F3016M-19: Standard Test Method for Surrogate Testing of Vehicle Impact Protective Devices at Low Speeds

- United Kingdom:
  - British Standards Institute:
    - BS EN 12767:2019 - Passive safety of support structures for road equipment - requirements and test methods
    - BSI PAS 170-1:2017 - Vehicle Security Barriers. Low Speed Impact Testing. Trolley Impact Test Method for Bollards

- International:
  - International Organization for Standardization (ISO), International Workshop Agreement
    - ISO/IWA-14 – Vehicle Security Barriers

While most vehicle impacts to retail storefronts and community care buildings are unintentional, they remain a threat to the people inside these buildings and to the ongoing operations of the practice(s) within. Proper bollard selection, layout, and installation is a solid strategy to mitigate this persistent threat.

3.4 Maintenance

Demonstrating that your organization and its staff care about the appearance of your facility can help deter criminal activity. A poorly maintained exterior sends the message that no one cares about what is happening outside. This is a potential invitation to others to loiter or commit crime on the property. A well-maintained exterior sends the opposite message- that the site and staff care and are vigilant about what's happening outside.

Some simple ways to maintain a site's exterior are to:

- Keep landscaping neat and well-trimmed. Landscaping should not obstruct the ability of people outside to see other people, vehicles, and other activity around them.
- Landscaping surrounding the perimeter of parking lots, walkways and around dumpster areas should not exceed 2 feet/.6 meters in height with a minimum depth of at least 4 feet/1.22 meters.
- Keep tree canopies high from the ground to keep them from blocking clear views of the area. Ensure that trees don't obstruct light fixtures.
- Keep bushes low to maintain good visibility outside. Remove bushes in the immediate vicinity of exterior doors and dumpster areas to prevent them from being used as a hiding place for a potential assailant.
- Ensure trash and other debris are regularly and promptly cleaned up.
- Address any vandalism, such as graffiti as soon as it happens.
- Utilize clear, well-placed signage outside that identifies the owner of the property and that warns against trespassing and illegal parking.

3.5 Exterior Access Control

3.5.1 Overview

The exterior perimeter of a community care site consists of the grounds, parking areas, and exterior of the building. Access controls at the exterior perimeter of a community care site helps ensure that legitimate users can easily enter the property while deterring and/or detecting non-legitimate users.

3.5.2 Fencing

Fencing around a community care site is not always feasible as these sites may be in a storefront setting, multi-tenant building, or a leased facility. However, when a standalone building is owned by the organization or when lease conditions permit, fencing can be a good way to enhance perimeter security.

In most cases, fencing will serve to limit access points onto the property during business hours to legitimate vehicle and pedestrian entry points. Funneling vehicle and pedestrian traffic through designated fence openings can help with monitoring of who is entering the site. This can also help deter criminal activity. Someone thinking of committing a crime may realize that their likelihood of detection is greater and escape routes are limited by fencing. If there is a need to prevent access to the site after hours due to high crime risk and/or illegal parking issues, locking gates may be installed across vehicle and pedestrian entrances to provide additional access controls.

3.5.3 Fencing Considerations

There are several considerations to keep in mind when deciding what type of fencing to use. Each organization is different and the crime risks facing each site can vary widely. Balancing the need for security can sometimes conflict with the mission of the organization. For example, a community care site may be located in a high-crime area to serve the community's most vulnerable populations. Installing a six-foot-tall fence around the perimeter of the center may conflict with the desired public perception that the center is safe and open to all in need.

Here are some issues to consider when it comes to fencing around a community care facility:

- **Crime risk:** An above average crime risk level may not be an immediate trigger for fencing. Consider the history of criminal incidents in the immediate area surrounding the facility and on the property.
- **Public perception:** Closing off exterior property access points at a facility located adjacent to or within the residential neighborhood it serves may send a message to the community that they are not welcome or trusted.
- **Fencing type:** A chain-link fence is not very aesthetically pleasing and may look more like an industrial site than a medical facility. Wrought-iron fencing is more visually pleasing but is expensive and requires more maintenance. Fencing that obscures the ability for staff to see out of the property and for the public or police to see into the property may increase the overall risk of crime at the site. Ultimately, the type of fence selected must meet the needs and budget of the organization.
- **Fencing specifications:** The risk of crime at the site should dictate the overall specifications of the fencing. However, fencing should be a minimum of 4 feet, extending to 6 feet for higher security applications in the US. In Canada and Europe, minimum fence heights are often 1 meter with higher security applications using up to 2-meter-high fences. However, in Australia, Singapore, and other countries, a 1.8-meter fence is the tallest height permitted. It's important to understand fencing regulations in your country and local area prior to installing anything.

In high-crime areas, fencing should be designed to be difficult to climb and cut. Barbed wire or concertina wire are rarely used to deter climbing due to their poor aesthetics and public perception impacts. The fence line should be inspected on a regular basis to identify areas where it may have been cut or damaged. Holes and other damage to the fence should be repaired promptly.

- **Gate considerations:** If you install locked limited-access gates or emergency-exit only gates for staff to use during business hours, the gates should have the following features:

  - Self-closing hinges to ensure that the gate consistently closes and fully latches/locks after opening.

  - A strong, solid metal barrier surrounding the interior handle, crash bar, and/or release button to prevent someone from reaching through the fence to open it.

  - An exterior card reader, numeric keypad, or keyed lock to limit access into the site.

3.5.4 Doors, Roof Hatches, and Windows

Perimeter doors are the first line of defense against unauthorized entry into a building, suite, or area. Typically, the front or main entrance door will be open to patients and others entering during business hours while the staff entrance(s) is locked with a key or card access. Anyone can walk through the main entrance of most community care sites, so internal layers of security are important during normal operating hours.

Most commercial grade, non-public exterior doors are made of steel with no window or a small to medium size window. In a suite located within a commercial building, these doors vary widely in quality and security, but are typically constructed of solid wood with or without a window. Usually, the most vulnerable door on the perimeter of a building or suite is the main entrance door(s). For aesthetic purposes, this door is usually composed of a large glass panel(s) surrounded by a metal frame. After hours, this door may be a target for unauthorized entry as it presents a path of least resistance for an intruder.

The roof hatch on a commercial building is often forgotten about as a possible point of entry for a burglar. This is especially true for single-story buildings, where climbing the building can be easier thanks to nearby dumpsters, trees, or other natural ladders.

The level of security needed for exterior perimeter doors varies depending on the level of risk in the area surrounding the site. The following elements should be in place for any community care site regardless of risk level:

- **Main Entrance Door(s):** Traditional hinged doors should be equipped with keyed, commercial-grade mortise locksets, at minimum. Sliding doors should be equipped with a hook bolt as turning off the door motor does not provide adequate security against intrusion.

A hook bolt slides vertically into place upon turning the key in the lock cylinder and "hooks" onto the inside of the door frame. This prevents the door from being forcefully slid open. For double doors, an astragal - usually a strip of metal – should be used to seal the gap between the doors to reduce the opportunity for unauthorized access by activating the crash bars.

- **Employee Entrance Door(s):** Employee entrance doors should be equipped with a keyed, commercial-grade mortise lockset, at minimum. Ideally, these doors should be equipped with an electronic lock and a card reader. This will help ensure that only authorized persons access these doors. Further, these doors should have a recessed or armored surface mounted door switch monitor (DSM) installed on them that are connected to a monitored building alarm system.

A solid employee entrance door should be equipped with a door scope to allow employees to see if anyone is outside the door before exiting. A door scope is similar to a traditional peephole but allows for a wide field of view (168-degrees) and is viewable up to 7-feet (2.1 meters) from the interior of the door. This helps encourage employees to use the scope before exiting. In contrast, a traditional peephole requires that employees place their eye close to the door and is less likely to be used. Door scopes should always be designed to prevent people outside from looking in.

Only authorized personnel who open, close, or service the facility (i.e.- cleaning service) should have employee entrance, perimeter door keys and/or card access authorization. Keys should be tracked upon issuance and return. If a key goes missing or is not returned by a former employee or service worker, the perimeter doors should be re-keyed.

- **Emergency Exits:** If a door is designated as an emergency exit only, it should not have a handle on the outside or an accessible lock cylinder. The door should be equipped with an audible alarm installed on it to alert staff when it has been opened. Further, these doors should have a recessed or armored surface mounted door switch monitor (DSM) installed on them that is connected to a monitored building alarm system.

  o Note: Staff are often their own worst enemies regarding emergency exit doors. They prop emergency exit doors open when going out to smoke or to grab lunch, leaving the door vulnerable to unauthorized entry. Evidence of a door that is frequently propped open is easy to spot: a large rock, stick, or wedge can usually be found immediately inside or outside the door. In some cases, frequent propping may indicate the need to add a legitimate means to re-enter the building through an exit door, such as a keyed lock or card access.

- **Roof Hatch:** The roof hatch should be always locked from the inside with a padlock affixed to the latch mechanism. The hatch should be equipped with a contact switch connected to a monitored building alarm system.

- **Windows:** In some facilities, exterior windows can be opened- presenting a way for someone to gain access either during or after business hours. Windows accessible from the ground are the most vulnerable, but windows on the second floor may also be vulnerable to access via a nearby tree, dumpster, or features on the building that form a natural ladder. If windows are opened during the day, staff should ensure that they are closed and locked when locking up the facility at night.

Depending on the risk level of the surrounding area and level of exposure to possible vandalism or intrusion, windows may need additional protection. There are two primary ways to add protection to windows: protective laminate/overlay and/or alarm monitoring:

- Protective Film: A protective film can be applied to existing windows to hold the window together if someone tries to smash it with an object to gain entry. The idea behind protective film is to delay an intruder and increase the likelihood that they will be detected. The level of protection afforded by protective film varies widely- from protection against rocks or a hammer to high-powered firearms. The level of protection should be dictated by the risks faced by the facility.
- Alarms: The types of alarm sensors typically used to monitor windows are glass break sensors that detect breaking glass or an open window, respectively. Alarm sensors can also be used in conjunction with protective film to sound an alarm when a forced entry attempt is made on a window. Glass break sensors must be connected to a monitored building alarm system.

3.6 Electronic Security

3.6.1 Overview

Electronic security is an important measure to have in place as part of a layered approach to security. As with any security measures, the type, level, and deployment of electronic security at a community care facility should be aligned with its overall security risk level.

For purposes of this section, electronic security consists of security cameras and recorders, card access and electronic locking systems, duress systems, and building alarm systems.

It's important that multi-site community care organizations and/or those connected to a larger hospital/healthcare system align electronic security systems and platforms whenever possible. Oftentimes, as community care sites are leased or purchased, the security systems already in place are adopted. This leads to security systems of varying quality at each site operating on different platforms that are often unable to integrate with one another. These systems may all require different vendors to service them as well.

Further, when card access platforms are not aligned across sites, there can be long-term operational and security impacts. Designated staff at each site end up maintaining their respective card access databases, sometimes poorly. This can lead to former personnel and contractors maintaining access to the building long after they have left. Also, staff floating between sites must carry multiple access cards or credentials for each location.

Lastly, electronic security systems must be maintained to be effective. Camera systems and card access systems need to have regular software and firmware updates through support agreements and licensing fees must be paid. Even simple building alarm systems must be regularly tested and receive preventative maintenance to function properly. Without proper maintenance, the systems may fail when they are needed most and may also be exposed to cyber threats.

3.7 Security Cameras

3.7.1 Overview

Security cameras play an important role as one of the several layers of security on the exterior of a community care site. The value of security cameras lies in the video they record for later review since security cameras at these sites are typically not monitored. Recorded video can help with investigations into incidents such as vehicle break-ins, slip and fall accidents, vehicle accidents, violent crime, and more.

When it comes to security cameras, there is a common misconception that they prevent and/or mitigate violence. The truth is that there is little to no research supporting this idea (Cameron et al., 2008; Piza et al., 2019).

However, security cameras have been found to prevent property crime, particularly in parking lots. The deterrent effect of these cameras in parking lots and other settings is dependent on the system being actively monitored and interventions following criminal activity detection (Cameron et al., 2008; Piza et al., 2019).

Security cameras should be deployed on the exterior of community care buildings when feasible. However, more effective exterior security layers outlined within this section, such as lighting, should be prioritized before installing cameras.

3.7.2 Camera Placement

At minimum, security cameras should be placed on the exterior of the community care facility to view the following areas:

- Exterior of the main entrance(s)
- Exterior of the employee entrance(s)
- Parking areas and sidewalks adjacent to the building
- Other parking areas

3.7.3 Camera Selection

Selecting the right cameras for the exterior of the facility is critically important. One way to help ensure the right cameras are selected is to engage a qualified, reputable professional security integrator company. Security integrators specialize in installing, merging, and maintaining building alarms, card access systems, and security camera systems.

Here are some key considerations when selecting exterior cameras:

- Always use commercial-grade cameras and never off-the-shelf residential cameras for longevity, serviceability, and secure design.
- Cameras should be designed for outdoor use (i.e.- weather proof)
- Vandal-resistant cameras should be used in locations that are accessible from the ground.
- Low light capabilities are important outdoors. Some cameras have invisible illumination built in (i.e.- infrared), while others have very low light sensitivity.
- Choose network cameras that transmit data through ethernet cables instead of legacy coaxial cable-based cameras. Network cameras enable enhanced features such as being powered over ethernet (PoE) cabling, higher quality images, and video analytics.
- For wide open areas like parking lots, consider using a multi-sensor camera, which enables multiple views of a wide area within a single housing.
- Ensure that cameras are not mounted too close to a light fixture that can cause glare.

3.7.4 Video Recording

Recording exterior video camera footage can be accomplished through an on-site network video recorder (NVR) or a cloud-based recording solution. Most community care sites utilize an on-site network video recorder. However, several companies now offer cloud-based recording, which may be more convenient and affordable for smaller organizations. Cloud-based recording removes the need to house and maintain a network video recording device on-site. This type of recording is subscription based and fees depend on the number of cameras streaming and amount of storage required.

Security cameras should be recording on a 24/7 basis with a minimum retention time of 30 days recording. The network video recorder should be set to record a minimum of 15 frames per second to capture sufficient images- particularly of objects in motion (IPVM, 2021). Video retention time can be increased by setting the video recorder to only record on motion. This means that the recorder only stores video when a connected camera detects a change (motion) in the scene it's monitoring.

3.7.5 Video Monitoring

Live monitoring of exterior security cameras in the community care setting is uncommon. If there are security personnel on-site, they may passively monitor video, but it's unlikely to be their primary focus. The same goes for video that is transmitted to a security operations center (SOC) when the site is part of a larger healthcare system.

Community care sites located in higher crime areas with a history of issues on the exterior of the facility may want to consider "remote guarding" services. These services are offered through a variety of vendors in the US and across the globe. Typically, a remote guarding vendor utilizes video analytics to identify when people and vehicles are loitering on property or when other issues are occurring. The remote guard can then contact police to respond and/or utilize loudspeakers (if installed/permitted) to "talk down" the person(s) in question. Talk down refers to verbal intervention warning to the person that the police are coming and to stop what they are doing and leave.

There are also other remote monitoring services that focus on the threat of firearms. One example of such a company is ZeroEyes™, which remotely monitors live video feeds from sites using video analytics that can detect visible firearms. When the analytics detect a firearm, the images are sent to a trained video operator, who quickly confirms whether there is a real firearm threat. A confirmed threat results in the operator contacting police and the site leadership/security team to alert them.

3.8   Card Access System

A card access system is a good way to control access at the exterior of a community care building or suite. This system utilizes a device located at a locked door that can read information from a credential (e.g.- an employee identification card). Once the credential is validated by the card access system, the electronic lock on the door unlocks to grant access.

Card access systems provide a greater ability to control who can access the facility and when they can access it. They also provide an audit trail of who entered the building and when they entered. Unlike a physical key, a person's credential can be quickly turned off if it is lost or stolen or if an employee or contractor is no longer authorized to enter the building.

Credentials for card access systems come in a variety of shapes and sizes including, but not limited to, key fobs, photo identification cards, and mobile credentials hosted on a smartphone. The level of security provided by these credentials can vary from basic to highly secure and encrypted.

Typically, card access does not need to be deployed on all exterior doors to the facility or suite. Only the doors regularly accessed by staff should be equipped with card access capabilities. Examples include the primary employee entrance, the service entrance, and the entrance located near an outdoor break area. All other doors, such as emergency exit doors, shouldn't be regularly used by staff and don't require card access.

It's important that all exterior doors are accessible only with a tightly controlled key. No one except key leadership should have this key as it can bypass the card access system and allow access into non-card access doors.

The card access system database must be regularly updated by a designated person(s) to ensure that people who no longer need access are removed from the system. An employee or contracted cleaning staff person who has been terminated or transferred should have their access privileges turned off as soon as possible to prevent unauthorized access into the building. Further, card access privileges should be controlled by time when possible, to prevent unauthorized employees or certain service personnel from entering the building after business hours. Ultimately, the card access system is only as secure as the database used to grant access privileges.

3.8.1 Lockdown Capabilities

A card access system can be utilized to enable a building or suite to rapidly lock down the doors if there's an external threat. Examples of an external threat include an active shooter in the area or a patient who has threatened to come to the facility to harm staff. To enable a lockdown, any door that is unlocked during business hours needs to be equipped with a minimum of an electronic lock connected to the card access system. Further, some doors, such as a sliding glass door at the main entrance, may need to be manually locked even after being electronically locked. Sliding doors can often be manually forced open from outside if they are not mechanically and electronically locked.

The fastest way to enable a quick lockdown of the facility is to have a physical lockdown button located in an area accessible to authorized staff, such as the reception desk. If a lockdown capability is enabled, staff at the facility must be trained in when and how to activate a lockdown. Staff should be empowered to lock down the facility if there's an imminent external threat to their safety and the safety of patients.

CHAPTER 4

Interior Physical Security Measures

4.1 Overview

Interior physical security measures help keep staff and patients safe during regular operating hours. They control the flow of patient traffic, provide protection for staff, and keep medication secure, among other benefits. These measures typically consist of locking doors and containers, security cameras, duress/panic alarms, and protective elements integrated into the interior environment.

In a typical community care site, the layers of physical security start at the lobby/waiting area, then progress into to other interior areas, such as medication rooms, storage areas, labs, utility closets, offices, and exam rooms.

To be effective, each layer of the interior security plan needs to be thoughtfully planned and designed to work together to provide protection. Further, staff must be trained on and understand the importance of interior security measures. A practice can have thousands of dollars' worth of security layers in place, but if an employee props open a locked door, the safety of the practice is immediately compromised.

This section walks through the most common security layers that should be in place within a community care site.

4.2 Check-In/Waiting Area

The first point of contact between a patient arriving at a community care site and staff occurs at the check-in/waiting area. The staff working in this area are often the first to encounter the frustration, anxiety, or anger of patients arriving for their appointments. Therefore, it's critical that this area supports the safety and security of staff and patients.

The following layers of security should be in place within any check-in/waiting area:

1. <u>Locked door(s) between the waiting and treatment areas.</u> A numeric code (cypher) operated lock or card reader are the most common ways to secure these doors. Also, the receptionist

at the front desk should have the ability to remotely grant access to the door using a release button or card reader at the desk. It's important that the lock on the door is easy and convenient to operate. Staff are more likely to prop open a door that is difficult to open. Card readers are easier to use than cypher locks for frequently used doors.

If there is a door to the treatment area behind the reception desk, it should be secured with a card reader. This is especially true if unauthorized persons can easily access the rear of the reception desk.

2. <u>A deep and tall enclosed reception/check-in desk.</u> There are several considerations when it comes to the first point of patient contact at the reception desk within a community care site:

   a. The front desk should ideally be four feet (1.2 meters) tall and four feet (1.2 meters) deep. The idea here is that the height and the depth of the desk combined help to keep someone from easily reaching over or jumping over the desk to harm staff.

   b. The desk should be fully enclosed to keep unauthorized persons from entering. A fully enclosed desk establishes a continuous perimeter around staff to prevent public access to the reception area. This means that publicly accessible entry doors to the desk area should be locked. Knee-height doors are useless as access control measures for a reception desk and should be replaced with full-height doors. An entry door to the desk located within the staff-only interior area of the practice is ideal.

   c. Adding a clear barrier across the entire opening of the desk is another means to provide protection against physical threats. Lexan™ or shatter resistant laminated glass can be used to provide enhanced protection from patient violence. These clear barriers should be installed in a way that balances staff safety with the need for communication and unimpeded interaction. Countertop to ceiling barriers will impede communication, leading to frustration on both sides of the glass and send the message that the practice is unsafe. If barriers that were installed for infection control during COVID-19 remain in place, they are likely not designed for security purposes and should be replaced with a more secure option.

   d. Staff behind the desk should be seated on elevated task chairs with footrests that place them at eye level with approaching persons. When staff are seated in a lower position and approaching patients are standing, patients are looking down on them. This can lead to patients subconsciously feeling superior to staff and staff feeling vulnerable or inferior to them.

It's important to note that in most countries, there are accessibility laws that require a portion of the counter to be of lower height and reduced depth. These areas, which can present a jump-over or reach-over risk to reception staff can also be protected with Lexan™ or shatter-resistant laminated glass. It's important to understand the specific requirements for accessibility in your region and to research and implement these in the design of the reception desk. Regional references include, but are not limited to, the Americans with Disabilities Act (ADA), Accessible Canada Act (ACA), Equality Act of 2010, and European Accessibility Act (EAA).

3. <u>Secure cash storage.</u> Cash is used less frequently by most patients who now prefer debit/credit cards and other electronic payment methods. However, cash collected for co-payments should be secured in a locked cashier drawer accessible only to reception and other authorized staff. The cashier drawer should be bolted to a sold surface, such as a counter. If a cash box is used instead of a purpose-built cashier drawer, the cash box should be bolted or screwed onto a solid surface as well.

4. <u>Diversions for patients.</u> Adequate diversions in the waiting room are helpful to keep patients occupied while waiting. If patients have nothing to do but stare at a clock on the wall waiting for their appointment, their anxiety and frustration may increase, leading them to become upset. Examples of diversions include available Wi-Fi with clearly visible and easy instructions for access, magazines, practice literature, coloring books and crayons for kids, and a television with calming programming. Avoid allowing access to change the channel or volume on the television. Utilize closed captioning when appropriate to eliminate television noise altogether. In larger community care sites, offering centralized vending machines, or a small café are both effective ways to keep patients happy while they are waiting for their appointments.

5. <u>White noise.</u> A quiet practice means that patients in the reception area can overhear the conversations between staff and patients. Patients provide identifying information which can be overheard by others, risking confidentiality. Soft, low volume music playing in the reception/waiting area, or a white noise machine operating can both help to muffle conversations at the reception desk.

4.3 Treatment Area

The main treatment area of a typical community care site includes numerous exam rooms, nurse and physician work areas, a lab, and supply/storage areas. These areas and their respective security measures are discussed below:

1. <u>Exam rooms</u>. These rooms make up most of the treatment area and should be designed with staff safety in mind. Whenever possible, the exam table and patient seating should be

placed furthest from the door to the room. The clinician work area(s) in the room should be closest to the door. This design makes it easier for staff to quickly leave the room if a patient attempts to assault them. Further, any items, such as sharps, and valuable/portable electronics should be secured/removed to prevent access and/or theft by patients.

2. <u>Supply/storage and lab areas</u>. The doors to rooms where medications, supplies, sharps, etc. are stored are often left unlocked or propped open for staff convenience. However, this leaves them vulnerable to access by unauthorized people. These rooms should be equipped with a storeroom function lock, which prevents the door from being left in an unlocked position and requires a key for entry. If the room is used frequently, make it easy for staff to access by installing a card reader or numeric code operated lock. The more inconvenient it is to access the room, the more likely staff will prop the door open. Pneumatic door closers should be utilized on these doors to ensure they close and lock after staff leave.

3. <u>Nurse and physician work areas</u>. When nurse and physician work areas are exposed to patients in the practice, they should have two means of egress to allow staff to quickly exit when they feel threatened. Further, there should be at least one panic/duress button in the work area to allow staff to discreetly summon security and/or police assistance in an emergency. In larger work areas, additional, conveniently located panic/duress buttons should be installed. Work areas enclosed within a room should also have sufficient panic/duress alarms installed. The room should be secured with a locked door controlled by a card reader or numeric code operated lock.

4.4 Emergency Shelter Room(s)

An emergency shelter room within a practice is a location where staff can shelter-in-place if needed during a violent event as they wait for police and/or security to arrive. Depending on the size of the facility, more than one of these rooms may be needed to ensure they are quickly accessible and can accommodate sufficient staff. Keep in mind that not everyone will go to the safe room during a security emergency – some staff may barricade themselves into their current room or evacuate. It should be easy for staff to identify the safe room, but difficult for a non-staff member to identify the room. Think about changing the color of the room number on the door to a bright color or adding a discreet marking to help staff identify the room. All staff should know where the room is, and it should be readily accessible to them. The basic elements of any safe room are as follows:

1. A solid, locking door - ideally equipped with a deadbolt.

2. No windows on the door or in the room to shield occupants from view. Ideally, the room should have solid cinderblock or brick walls to help protect occupants from bullets. An X-Ray room can be a good safe room location due to the lead lining in the walls.

3. A phone and/or a panic alarm monitored by an alarm monitoring center inside to allow occupants to summon help if they do not have their cell phones or cell reception.

These rooms aren't just for emergencies; they are functional rooms in the facility that double as emergency shelter rooms.

4.5 Building Alarm System

A building alarm system is a good way to add a layer of security during and after operating hours. The alarm system should be installed, maintained, and regularly tested by a qualified professional and monitored by a properly certified 24/7 alarm monitoring center. A typical building alarm system consists of a control panel, keypad, door switch monitors, motion sensors, glass break sensors, alarm sounder, and system interruption sensors. Building alarm systems may also include duress alarms and water sensors. Here's a breakdown of each component:

- **Control panel:** The control panel is the brains of the system and there may be more than one panel required depending on the size of the system and the facility. The control panel is connected to an alarm monitoring center through a telephone line or network connection. Some systems utilize a cellular connection as a primary or secondary form of connection. The control panel should have a battery backup to ensure that building protection is maintained during a power failure. It should also be equipped with a tamper alarm so that opening the door to the panel causes it to go into alarm.
- **Keypad:** The keypad controls the alarm system. It is typically located closest to the employee entrance. The keypad is most often used to place the system into "armed" status to monitor and protect the building when it's not occupied and into "disarmed" status when the building is occupied. Arming and disarming is typically done using a numeric code. The alarm code should never be written on the keypad or anywhere else near it (yes- this really happens).
- **Door switch monitors:** Electronic door switch monitors (DSMs) should be installed on all exterior perimeter doors and roof hatches to detect whether a door is open or closed. DSMs should be recessed into the door and frame. If they must be surface mounted, DSMs should be protected with armored (metal surround) sensors and cabling to prevent tampering.
- **Motion Sensors:** Motion sensors utilize passive infrared (PIR) technology that detects body heat rather than just any movement in the building. These should be deployed to monitor main hallways, common areas, and lobbies. The idea behind motion sensors is threefold: 1) to serve as the primary point of detection when someone has entered through an unprotected window or may have remained in the building after closing; 2) to detect the current location of someone who is in the building to help the police find them; 3) to validate for police that someone is in the building following a perimeter door alarm activation.

- **Glass Break Sensors:** Glass break sensors detect the sound of breaking glass. These sensors can be prone to false alarm from loud sounds after hours and are typically deployed near each ground level window or set of windows.
- **Alarm Sounder:** An alarm sounder is a loudspeaker that transmits a loud siren sound inside the building to scare off an intruder. Alarm sounders are not a necessary part of a burglar alarm system as they don't always deter intruders. A silent alarm may be more likely to aid police in apprehending the intruder.
- **System Interruption Sensors:** System interruption sensors are a critical part of the building alarm system. These sensors "supervise" the system and report unusual conditions to the alarm monitoring center through the control panel. Typical situations that are monitored are power loss, panel tamper, and device health. Device health can include low battery alerts for wireless devices, low battery alert for the control panel, and a disconnect between the control panel and a motion sensor, door switch monitor (DSM), or another device.

4.5.1 Additional Components

Additional components can be added to a basic building alarm system to expand the functionality. Two common additional components are as follows:

- **Duress Alarms:** A duress, or panic, alarm is typically a button or pull switch that is used by an employee to indicate that they need emergency police assistance. Most often, duress alarms are hardwired to a discreet button under a desk. They may also be more visibly mounted on a wall in an exam room. Duress alarms can also be wireless. Wireless alarms are used when an employee might need assistance, but they are not near a wired duress button. The alarms usually transmit a signal to a nearby receiver that activates an alarm at the control panel.

   There are three common issues with traditional wireless duress alarms: 1) they are left in areas not easily accessible to staff, like a drawer or cabinet; 2) batteries are not proactively maintained; 3) they give responding police only a general idea of where the employee is located, since the transmitter may cover a wide area.

   However, there are newer, more effective wireless panic/duress systems that address these issues and more that should be explored when considering using traditional wireless duress buttons.

- **Water Sensors:** Water sensors or "water bugs" as they are sometimes called, monitor floors for water. These can be a great addition to an existing alarm system to detect flooding in a basement, mechanical room, mop sink room, etc. An undetected leak can cause serious damage to a community care site, particularly when undetected overnight or during a weekend.

4.5.2 System Codes and Response

It's important that only staff or contractors with a legitimate need to arm and disarm the system have the code to the alarm system. Each authorized person should be issued their own unique alarm code so that system activity can be audited by individual employee. There should never be one code for everyone to share. Codes must be disabled in a timely fashion upon an employee or contractor permanently leaving the facility.

When an alarm is activated after hours, an employee should never serve as a first responder to the building. If an employee must respond to a site to help police gain access to the building, they should only enter at the direction of, and under the protection of, the police.

CHAPTER 5

Site Operational Security

5.1 Overview

Beyond physical security, every community care site must incorporate a minimum level of security into their daily operations. Weaving security into site operations won't feel like additional work for staff and leadership if it's done right. The operational security measures outlined below, except for establishing a code word, are all proactive. Each of these measures should be supported by a policy/procedure. Further, staff should be trained on each policy/procedure initially and on a reasonable cadence (i.e., annually and via scenario-based micro-learning activities).

5.2 Opening and Closing Procedures

Opening and closing times at community care sites can possibly expose staff to external risks. At most sites, there is typically one person who enters the building or suite at the start of the day and disarms the building alarm system. At the end of the day, there is typically more than one person leaving the building. Opening and closing time procedures should incorporate reasonable security measures to keep staff safe. For example, procedures should include instructing staff not to approach the building during opening time or exit the building during closing time if they feel unsafe based on their observations of a suspicious person or vehicle. Instead, staff should trust their gut and call police for assistance.

5.3 Cleaning Service

Cleaning companies typically service community care sites after business hours. The cleaning service staff should be instructed to always keep the building perimeter locked while inside. If possible, the building alarm should be set to "stay" mode (motion sensors off) while inside so that any unauthorized entry attempts are detected. Lastly, cleaning staff must alarm the building prior to leaving at the end of the night.

5.4 Pre-Appointment Communications

Pre-appointment reminders and other communications are a great way to minimize frustration for patients prior to their arrival. For example, many practices now provide the links to forms that need to be filled out for the appointment instead of handing the patient a clipboard filled with paperwork upon arrival. This effort streamlines the patient's registration and check-in process and minimizes any surprises for them. Pre-appointment reminders can also inform patients about where to park when they arrive. This information can reduce patient frustration and the chances that patients will be late for appointments. While not every patient will read their pre-appointment communications, those that do will most likely experience increased visit satisfaction and less frustration.

5.5 Wait Times

Patient frustration can be mitigated by communicating wait times to them in advance. For example, in an urgent care setting, providing the approximate wait time on the website for the location can help set expectations for patients. The same wait time can be displayed immediately inside the urgent care lobby by the check-in desk. In a primary care practice, a simple whiteboard can display the doctor's name and their status (i.e., on time or delayed). This same information can be verbally communicated to patients upon check-in. The key here is to overcommunicate, set expectations from the start, and to update patients if anything changes while they are waiting. These efforts can help mitigate patient frustration caused by the expectation of a quick visit that is met with the reality of a twenty-minute delay.

5.6 Diversions

Diversions for patients are methods to keep them from focusing on the wait time. These diversions don't need to be elaborate or costly. For example, simply providing the password in a visible area of the waiting room for the public Wi-Fi can ensure that patients can use their smartphones for a diversion. A fish tank in a pediatrician's office can help keep parents happy (because their kids are occupied) while they wait. When selecting diversions, try to provide more than one option and ensure that the diversions are appropriate for the patient population.

5.7 Code word

A code word or phrase is a way for staff to discreetly communicate that they need help with a potential safety/security risk. The code word/phrase should be established and communicated to all staff with regular reminders. The word or phrase should be something uncommon that fits within the context of regular daily operations. For example, a physician might say to a nurse, "Sarah, can you see if that fax came in from Dr. Gold?" Dr. Gold is the code word here.

Upon hearing the code word/phrase, the nurse should know what to do next. This could mean that the nurse helps make an excuse to get the physician out of the room or that they call the police. Either way, every staff member should know what to do when they hear the code word/phrase. A code word/phrase is useless if staff don't know what do to when they hear it.

5.8 See Something, Say Something

A "see something, say something" culture should be established at the site. All staff should be encouraged to report any concerning behaviors, communications, and/or observations to site leadership and/or security. It's vitally important that staff know to trust their gut instincts when they feel unsafe and report it immediately.

See something, say something is not just for front desk staff, but for everyone at the site. For example, a physician who feels that their patient may be harboring a grudge against them for a recent procedure outcome should report it. Staff should know who to report issues to and how to do it. Reporting should be regularly and strongly encouraged. All reported issues should be investigated, appropriate actions taken to address the issue, and the results reported back to the staff member making the report.

5.9 Conclusion

Nearly all the site security operations elements listed in this section cost nothing to implement. Further, all of them can be incorporated into daily activities at the site. These daily practices not only help reduce patient frustration and stress, but they also increase patient satisfaction and staff safety. With less conflict happening between patients and staff, staff will also be happier. Meanwhile, the level of security at the site will be quietly enhanced in the background.

CHAPTER 6

Emergency Preparedness

6.1 Overview

There are a variety of emergency situations that can occur at community care sites. This section covers the essential security-related emergency situations that care sites should be prepared to handle. For each emergency scenario outlined below, there should be:

- A written policy and procedure
- A quick reference version of the policy and procedure readily available to staff
- Initial training for all staff
- Ongoing refresher training for all staff, including scenario-based micro-learning "drills"

It's also important to involve local first responder leadership to ensure they understand the site's plans. These leaders can also help determine whether these plans are realistic given their response time and other capabilities. Lastly, in an enterprise-level organization, policies and procedures written for enterprise hospitals are sometimes adopted by care sites. These policies and procedures should always be modified to fit the resources and limitations of each care site before being adopted by the site.

6.2 Emergency Notification Method

Every site should have the ability to quickly notify all staff in the practice of a security-related or other emergency. There are several ways to communicate quickly within a community care site:

- Mass notification system that uses a variety of means to notify staff: text, phone call, email desktop alert. This is best for very large sites and multi-site organizations.
- Overhead speaker/public announcement system.

- Intercom function on the internal phone system.
- An audible security alarm triggered by pressing a panic/duress alarm.
- Good old-fashioned yelling (for very small sites).

Regardless of the type of notification method, all staff should be trained on how and when they should alert site staff to an emergency. If notification relies on any type of technology (applies to all but yelling), the system used should be tested monthly to ensure it is functioning properly.

6.3 Essential Security-Related Emergency Plans

6.3.1 Active Shooter/Active Threat

While this is the rarest type of security-related emergency, it is also the scenario most community care site staff fear the most. An active shooter is defined by the FBI as "one or more individuals actively engaged in killing or attempting to kill people in a populated area. Implicit in this definition is the shooter's use of a firearm." (FBI, 2022). An active threat typically is defined in a similar manner, although the threat can be from any type of traditional or improvised weapon, such as a knife or a metal pole, respectively.

These events can unfold very quickly and often without warning. Most are over in a matter of minutes and end prior to the arrival of law enforcement. This is why it's important for site staff to be trained and prepared for this unlikely but dangerous threat.

While these events are frightening to think about, the likelihood of an active shooter or active threat situation unfolding inside of a community care site is quite low. However, the risk is not zero and the impact of such an event would be devastating to staff, patients, the organization, and its reputation.

In the United States, the threat of an active shooter is what many community care site employees fear most. However, preparing site staff for this threat can help everyone feel more empowered to respond. Here's the key elements needed to prepare community care sites for this potential threat:

- **Procedure:** Create a procedure for responding to an active shooter/active threat should be developed that follows the Run-Hide-Fight (or Defend) methodology is common in the United States, Canada, UK, Australia, and other countries. There are many different variations on this procedure. Ultimately, each organization should determine what methodology best fits for their situation. The selected methodology should be based on the advice of law enforcement and security experts.
- **Training:** Train your staff what to do in the event of an active shooter/active threat event. There are plenty of free online active shooter training videos available online but be sure to choose a video created by a recognized law enforcement agency. Review the training video to ensure that it is not presented in a way that would create unnecessary fear among staff.

Some videos use graphic imagery and language that can alarm viewers and make it harder for them to retain the key messages in the training. Utilize scenario-based micro-learning to keep training fresh.
- **Safe Rooms:** Identify locations where your staff can shelter-in-place. Selecting and equipping safe rooms is covered elsewhere in this manual.
- **Exits:** Ensure that all emergency exits are always accessible and that the doors are in good working order. In smaller practices, pathways to exit doors are sometimes obstructed by equipment and supplies. Further, seldom used exit doors may become difficult to open if they are not maintained properly. Accessible and functional emergency exits are essential for staff safety from fire and other emergencies as well.

6.3.2 External Threat

An external security threat could occur at any time. This could be a situation where a patient has called and is threatening to come to the site and commit an act of violence. It could also be a threat unrelated to the site like a violent criminal being sought by police in the area.

Here's the key elements needed to prepare community care sites for this potential threat:

- **Procedure:** Develop a procedure that outlines what is considered and external threat. Identify the steps to respond to such a threat and who is authorized to lock down the site. All staff should be empowered to quickly lock down the site without supervisor approval if there's an imminent threat. The procedure should also outline how to communicate with patients when a lockdown has occurred.

- **Training:** Ensure all staff receive initial and ongoing training to identify and respond to an external threat and that they know their role in locking down the site.

- **Lockdown:** The ability to quickly lock down the facility is essential to respond to an external security threat. Ideally, there should be a single button readily available to staff to lock all doors. For sites with a single-entry door, having the keys or other device needed to lock the door quickly available to staff is needed.

6.3.3 Violent Person

A violent person is someone who is being physically violent towards one or more people at the site or who appears to pose an imminent threat of physical violence. While less common in the community care setting, a patient, staff member, stranger, or an outsider with a personal relationship to someone at the site could act out violently.

Common types of violence in the community care setting are covered in more depth elsewhere within this manual. The emergency response focus here is on the imminent threat of physical violence and physical violence in progress. Here's the key elements that should be in place for this type of threat:

- **Procedure:** The violent person procedure should define physical violence and the imminent threat of physical violence. It should also outline options for staff response, methods to alert and get co-workers and patients to safety, how to summon police quickly (including panic alarms), and safe room/shelter-in-place locations.

- **Training:** Staff should receive initial and ongoing refresher training on the violent person procedure. As part of the training, all staff should be empowered to trust their instincts and summon help quickly if they feel there's an imminent threat of violence.

6.3.4 Conclusion

While there are a variety of emergency situations that can unfold in a community care site, these are the most essential security-related situations that staff should be prepared to handle. The ultimate key to preparing staff for such events is training and empowerment.

CHAPTER 7

Workplace Violence in the Community Care Setting

7.1 Types of Violence in the Community Care Setting

Patient violence in the community care setting typically takes the form of verbal abuse and threats. While less common in these settings, physical violence is always a possibility. In rare instances, physical violence can escalate to a deadly encounter.

7.1.1 Common Types of Violence in the Community Care Setting

1. **Verbal Abuse:** Verbal abuse in the community care setting is typically committed by patients. However, verbal abuse can come from anyone within or outside of the site. This type of violence involves threatening or abusive language towards staff and others, such as threats of harm to self or others, and racist, sexist, sexual, or otherwise demeaning and inappropriate language. This language is typically intended to place the person in imminent fear for their physical safety, intimidate or harass them.

2. **Threats:** Threats in the community care setting are also most often committed by patients. However, threats can come from current or former employees, visitors, family members of patients, strangers, and personal relations of staff. While threats can take the form of verbal or physical violence, they can also take the form of written communication through email, text, mail, and other formats. These threats may be communicated when the patient is in the care environment or after they have left. A threat can generally be defined as a statement or action that places another person in fear for their safety from physical harm.

7.1.2 Less Common Types of Violence in the Community Care Setting

1. **Physical Violence:** Patients are the most likely perpetrators of physical violence in the community care setting. However, physical violence can be perpetrated by anyone within or outside of a practice. Physical violence includes both assault and battery.

    a. Assault is placing someone in imminent fear of battery. This is often accomplished by actions such as assuming a fighting stance, pointing a finger in someone's face, or attempting to grab or strike someone with a fist or foot.

    b. Battery is making physical contact with someone without their consent in a way that is likely to cause bodily harm and may include punching, pinching, biting, kicking, pushing, and other actions.

        i. Sexual battery is generally defined as touching the intimate part of another person (buttocks, breasts, genitals), whether clothed or unclothed, against their will for the purpose of sexual arousal, sexual gratification, or sexual abuse.

2. **Domestic Violence:** Patients and staff in the community care setting may be in a domestic violence situation that can spill into the workplace. Healthcare staff face an elevated risk of domestic violence. A recent study found that 45% of healthcare workers in Australia had experienced domestic abuse- particularly female staff (McLindon et al., 2018). According to the US Department of Justice Office on Violence Against Women (OVW), domestic violence is defined as follows:

    "…a pattern of abusive behavior in any relationship that is used by one partner to gain or maintain power and control over another intimate partner. Domestic violence can be physical, sexual, emotional, economic, psychological, or technological actions or threats of actions or other patterns of coercive behavior that influence another person within an intimate partner relationship. This includes any behaviors that intimidate, manipulate, humiliate, isolate, frighten, terrorize, coerce, threaten, blame, hurt, injure, or wound someone." (Office of Violence Against Women, 2023).

3. **Stalking:** Stalking behaviors can be directed at patients and staff. These situations can arise from personal relationships outside of the community care setting or they can originate from within the practice. Stalking is generally defined as:

"...a course of conduct directed at a specific person that would cause a reasonable person to feel fear. Unlike other crimes that involve a single incident, stalking is a pattern of behavior...made up of individual acts that could, by themselves, seem harmless or noncriminal, but when taken in the context of a stalking situation, could constitute criminal acts" ("Stalking," 2021).

There are laws on the books in every state in the US against stalking that include the specific elements of the crime. In the UK, stalking crimes are primarily covered under the Protection from Harassment Act of 1997. In Australia, stalking crimes are contained within Section 13 under the Crimes (Domestic and Personal Violence Act) of 2007. Across the EU, most member states have enacted stalking laws.

7.1.3 Rare Types of Violence in the Community Care Setting

1. **Murder:** While murder is very rare in the community care setting, planning for extreme violence must still be considered. Murder is defined by the FBI Uniform Crime Reporting (UCR) Program as "...the willful (nonnegligent) killing of one human being by another" ("Murder," 2019, para. 1). Internationally, the World Health Organization's definition of murder/homicide is, "...the killing of a person by another with intent to cause death or serious injury, by any means. It excludes death due to legal intervention and operations of war" (Violence info – homicide 2023).

   Data on the number of murders in community care settings are difficult to come by at the international level, but in the US, there have been several instances of murders in the community care setting between 2022-2023:

   - On May 3, 2023, a medication seeking patient shot five people in an Atlanta medical building in waiting room, killing one and injuring four.

   - On July 11, 2023, a patient fatally shot his hand surgeon in an exam room in Tennessee in what was described as a targeted attack.

   - On June 1, 2022, a patient armed with a rifle killed his physician, a second physician, a receptionist, and another patient in Oklahoma. The patient, who had purchased the rifle just hours before the attack, blamed his physician for ongoing pain after back surgery.

   Despite these incidents, murder in the community care setting remains a rare occurrence-particularly considering the number of community care clinics in the US and across the globe and the millions of patients they treat every day.

2. **Rape:** Rape is also very rare in the community care environment. It is defined by the FBI Uniform Crime Reporting (UCR) Program as "...penetration, no matter how slight, of the vagina or anus with any body part or object, or oral penetration by a sex organ of another person, without the consent of the victim" ("Rape," 2019).

   While instances of rape are rare in the community care environment, there have been reported instances of rape at the hands of physicians entrusted to care for patients within the community care setting in the US. In 2023 alone, three separate physicians in Massachusetts have been accused by their patients of rape. In these cases, numerous patients have come forward with additional accusations after the news broke.

7.2 Violence Prevention & Mitigation in the Community Care Setting

7.2.1 Violence Risk Assessment

To understand the risk of violence in the community care setting, a violence risk assessment should be performed at each site and updated at least every two years. To assess a site's exposure to violence risk, there are several factors to consider. The general assessment process to identify violence risk is outlined below. Exposure to violence risks, the likelihood of events occurring, and the impact of those events identified in your assessment should drive prevention and mitigation measures.

1. <u>Interview site staff.</u> Staff can provide some of the best insights into violence risks present within and outside the facility. This is especially true given the serious underreporting of violence by healthcare staff – a trend that applies internationally. Be sure to interview both leadership and line staff from the front desk to clinical practice areas.

   When conducting interviews, look for common themes among staff and leadership that indicate shared concerns. Interviews can be conducted formally or informally. Typically, interviewing staff informally in their work area can help them feel more comfortable speaking about violence issues- especially if their colleagues are around. Employees in this setting may offer additional information that wouldn't otherwise be obtained in a formal, one-on-one or group interview.

2. <u>Look at past incidents and their frequency.</u> Has the site had previous incidents of staff being physically assaulted, threatened, or fearing for their safety? How often does it happen? Are incidents trending upwards, downwards or are they flat? How often are the police called to the site?

   As noted above, the violence underreporting plaguing hospitals is often worse at community care sites. Staff at these sites, often with little to no security support, feel that nothing will be done if they report violence. In community care settings that are part of a larger organization, staff often feel disconnected from the main hospital campus. This also leads staff to adopt a mindset that reporting won't trigger an investigation, response, or change, so they don't report. As noted previously, a better understanding of violence at the site may come from staff interviews vs. incident report data.

3. <u>Understand crime risk in the surrounding area.</u> The risk of crime in the area surrounding the facility can place staff and patients at risk of becoming victims of crime inside or outside the facility. There's a couple of ways to assess crime risk:

    a. Ask the local police department for the crime statistics for the community surrounding the site for the last three years or find it on their website.

    b. Purchase a professional crime risk report online that provides a better overall crime risk picture. These reports use more sophisticated formulas that consider actual crimes committed and the circumstances that can increase or decrease the likelihood of crime. There are two primary companies that provide these reports: CAP Index and SecurityGauge. Both companies provide reports for the US and Canada, while CAP Index also services the UK and Mexico.

4. <u>Examine patient and population mix.</u> Does the current or future patient mix or population create inherent risk for patients and/or staff? Examples include, but are not limited to, patients arriving in crisis, medication seeking patients, and vulnerable patients living in low socioeconomic conditions.

    When it comes to patient populations, a stable patient mix can help with predictability. For example, in a practice with long-term patients, like a family medicine practice, staff know most patients and their families very well. There's a known patient history and interactions are generally more predictable. However, if the patient population is more transient, like in an urgent care facility, staff may not know patients or their history at all. Patients may arrive in crisis for a variety of reasons, and that can increase unpredictability and risk.

    A single physician's patient population can even drive issues within a practice. At one of my previous client sites, a new physician brought a large population of medication seeking patients with him. These patients were calling the front desk and threatening reception desk and clinical staff and showing up without appointments demanding medications. When practice leadership heard these staff complaints and realized that new patients were driving to the suburban clinic from out-of-state just for prescriptions, they became suspicious and the physician was terminated from the practice.

5. <u>Think like an aggressor.</u> If you wanted to assault someone in the waiting area, treatment area, or parking lot, how would you do it? What would facilitate this assault? What would mitigate it? For example, if you wanted to grab the front desk receptionist, you'd probably reach over the counter at them. However, if the receptionist is behind a high, deep counter and the door to the reception area is locked, the likelihood of a successful attack is diminished.

6. <u>Conduct a penetration audit.</u> How secure is your treatment area against unauthorized access? Can someone gain access to your practice after hours? Can patients or trespassers gain access into employee only areas? Are doors left unlocked or propped open? More layers of protection against unauthorized entry means more protection afforded to staff and patients.

7.2.2 Violence Risk Assessment Analysis

Once you have gathered information through the violence risk assessment process, categorize the risks you identified by likelihood of occurrence, impact, and your preparedness for these risks. Example:

- What is the likelihood of a patient on staff assault occurring based on historical data/area crime risk/industry trends?

    ○ What would be the impact on people, assets, operations, and reputation?

    ○ What is level of preparedness for such an event or issue?

When scoring each of these categories, you can use a simple 1 to 5 scale. One is the lowest likelihood of occurrence, impact, and lowest level of preparedness. Five is the highest likelihood of occurrence, impact, and highest level of preparedness. This approach will help you to determine which risks require attention more urgently.

Note that preparedness is a mitigating factor. For example, a high level of preparedness (training) can help mitigate a very likely event (patient verbal abuse) with moderate impact (upset staff/minor operations disruption).

Results of the assessment should be documented, and appropriate leadership should keep track of actions taken to mitigate or prevent identified risks and when they were taken. Not only will this documentation serve as a point of accountability, but it can also be helpful with accrediting bodies, government/regulatory agencies, and to defend against inadequate security liability.

For multi-site community care operations, an initial violence risk assessment should be completed at each site. Multi-site community care findings should be compiled to identify risk commonalities among sites. These common risks can be used to formulate organization-wide improvements to mitigate known risks.

7.2.3 Violence Risk Assessment – External Consultants

When a more thorough and objective security risk assessment is desired, consider hiring a qualified healthcare security consultant. The consultant should have demonstrated expertise and credentials in healthcare security. Alternatively, local law enforcement may have the ability to conduct a general crime prevention survey of your site. However, law enforcement lacks specific healthcare security knowledge that is critical to understanding the unique risks within a care environment.

7.3 Essential Violence Prevention & Mitigation Measures

7.3.1 Overview

This section covers essential violence prevention and mitigation measures to address more common risks in the community care environment. For additional violence prevention and mitigation measures regarding patient violence, reference the Patient Violence Prevention and Mitigation Healthcare Security Field Manual.

7.3.2 Encourage Reporting

Encourage employees to report violent, threatening, concerning, or suspicious behavior by patients, co-workers, or others to their immediate supervisor, human resources, or security. Ideally, staff should also be able to file a report in a safety reporting system for documentation and follow-up. If possible, provide an anonymous reporting option as well to allow employees to report issues confidentially. Staff should also understand that they shouldn't hesitate to call the police whenever there's an imminent risk of violence.

7.3.3 Investigate Incidents and Support Victims of Violence

Every incident of violence in the community care setting should be investigated to determine: the root cause (if known) and/or events preceding the incident; who was impacted by the violence; and whether follow-up action is required. The investigation may be cursory or in-depth depending on the circumstances and severity of the incident. The investigation will likely be conducted by site leadership, but it is important that they collaborate with other stakeholders, such as security, human resources, risk management, and clinical leadership.

The victim(s) should be regularly updated on the status of the investigation to reassure them that the incident is being taken seriously. Consistent and transparent investigations can help encourage staff to report incidents more frequently, as the word will spread among them that reporting leads to follow-up.

Further, victims of violence require varying levels of support depending on the type of violence, whether there was a physical and/or psychological injury, and the level of actual and/or perceived future risk experienced by the victim. Support may include a referral to the Employee Assistance Program, assistance with filing criminal charges and/or obtaining a protective order, a follow-up by the victim's manager and/or human resources, a personalized safety plan, and more.

7.3.4 Support Employee Wellbeing

An employee assistance program (EAP) is a great way to support staff wellbeing. While most community care sites cannot offer an on-site EAP program, they are typically available remotely by phone and/or videoconference. An EAP helps to mitigate employee stressors related to experiencing violence. It can also help with life issues that can lead to employee violence by providing a relief valve and support.

7.3.5 Provide De-escalation Training

De-escalation training is frequently overlooked for community care sites. This is true even when community care sites are part of a healthcare enterprise. The importance of this training in an environment where the violence safety gap can range from a few minutes to more than ten minutes cannot be overstated.

A solid training program is the key to empowering staff to prevent escalation or to de-escalate volatile situations until help can arrive. When choosing a de-escalation program for the community care setting or evaluating the current one, here are some key considerations:

a. Select a program from recognized training provider that utilizes sound principles for both de-escalation and physical techniques. Programs developed in-house are not a good option from a variety of standpoints, especially when it comes to liability.

b. The program should be specifically tailored to the healthcare environment using a trauma-informed approach whenever possible.

c. Online training should be an option, especially since community care site staff don't have much time for training activities. Online courses should be broken into smaller chunks so that staff can pick away at lessons when they have time.

d. Physical skills training should always be conducted in person by a certified trainer.

e. The definition of workplace violence, types of workplace violence, national statistics, risk factors, situational awareness, and reporting procedures should be included in the course or through a supplemental course.

f. The program should utilize a tiered approach so that it can be rolled out to staff across the organization based on their risk level. Staff with direct patient care responsibilities and leaders who respond to escalating situations should generally have the highest level of training.

g. A train-the-trainer option should be available so that the organization can leverage its own instructors to teach the in-person portions of the course and sustain the training program.

Ongoing refresher training should happen at least twice a year, but annual refresher training is preferred.

Further, sites should leverage scenario-based micro-learning to keep staff safe between formal trainings. Micro-learning can be conducted by a member of site leadership or security with one or more staff members. This type of training is helpful for keeping staff skills related to violence prevention and mitigation fresh.

The importance of refresher training is illustrated by the Ebbinghaus forgetting curve and subsequent research into this phenomenon that found, "learners will forget on average 90% of material within 1 month" (Woolliscroft, 2020, p. 250). However, this research has also revealed that "…revisiting material at regular intervals, whether through presentations, electronic communication, or testing, enhances retention" (Woolliscroft, 2020, p. 257). To ensure that staff de-escalation skills and related violence prevention and mitigation skills stay front-of-mind, regular, bite-sized refresher opportunities are essential.

7.3.6 Plan in Advance for Concerning Patients

Safety preparations should be made prior to a patient's arrival whenever there is a concern that a patient may act out during their visit. Examples include patients who may react poorly to bad news (i.e., termination of care), those with a history of disruptive behavior, or patients who may act out violently.

Staff should discuss safety concerns about a patient with their supervisor as far in advance as possible. The supervisor should collaborate with other key leadership and the security team (if applicable) to determine whether the patient may pose a risk to staff or others. When needed, the leadership team should engage an external threat assessment professional to assess the potential risk posed by the patient. Any time there is a concern for imminent violence, the police should be called immediately for assistance.

The plan for the patient's visit should be based on the outcome of the patient risk assessment. Whenever possible, site leadership and staff should attempt to understand and mitigate any potential triggers or conflicts with the patient prior to their visit. This should ideally be accomplished through a pre-appointment secure videoconference or phone call. If the patient will be seen in person, ensure that all staff- from the front desk to clinicians- are aware of the patient visit plan and their role in the plan.

At times, the plan for the patient's visit may include a security or police detail. If utilized, the security or police detail officer should understand the plan for the patient's visit and what is expected of detail officer. Ideally, the detail officer should not be in uniform to avoid escalating the patient and/or raising concerns among other patients. Considerations and best practices for engaging external security services are detailed in Chapter 9.

After the patient visit, the care team and leadership should hold a debriefing to discuss the outcome. Further, a plan should be developed for future visits and patient care. This longer-term plan should establish ongoing safety protocols and triggers for upgrading or downgrading safety measures.

Lastly, if a patient's care with the site has been terminated, site leadership and staff must understand that this does not mean that the safety issues posed by the patient have been erased. In fact, the patient whose care was terminated may be triggered by the event. A long-term safety plan should be established to prevent and mitigate future issues with the patient.

7.3.7 Mitigate Firearms Risks

Firearms in healthcare facilities are a common concern- particularly in the US where gun ownership is constantly increasing. It's important to establish a written policy and procedure regarding firearms for community care sites. Once established, it's equally important to clearly communicate the policy to staff, patients, contractors, and anyone else with a relationship to the site. Regular and clear communications about your policy to patients prior to their arrival for an appointment will help to head off conflicts. Here are some considerations when developing the site's stance on firearms and implementing the policy:

- Decide whether the site will allow firearms and, if so, under what circumstances.
- Understand state laws regarding firearms and where they can and cannot be carried. A good way to understand these laws is through local police department leadership.
- Allowing firearms onsite can place staff, patients, and others at increased risk of serious injury or death. A patient or staff member may carry a firearm for personal protection and without the intent to harm someone. However, if a conflict erupts and the patient or staff member becomes angry, the firearm is immediately available and may be used to intimidate or harm others.
- If the practice will prohibit firearms, it's important to communicate this to patients before they arrive for an appointment. This can be done in appointment reminder communications and through other means. Heading off a conflict onsite is the goal here.
- Most community care sites will need to make an exception to their firearms policy for law enforcement officers carrying firearms while acting in an official capacity. If not, it is likely that conflict will arise when police are called to the site to assist with an issue.
- Installing signage on the entrance to each site that clearly states that firearms are prohibited is key to communicating a no firearms policy. Even if a patient states that they didn't know about the policy in advance, the signage is a clear reminder that firearms are prohibited.
- If firearms are permitted at the site, ensure that there is somewhere secure for patients to store them during their visit. Providing a secure lock box designed to hold firearms is

a helpful way to ensure that the patient feels comfortable securing their firearm on site during their visit. The only key to the lock box containing the firearm should be given to the patient to hold during their visit.
- Decide in advance whether the site will refuse service to someone who has a firearm and how staff will handle this. This is something that should be decided in advance and the proper response to this situation should be outlined in your policy and procedure regarding firearms and through a script for staff.
- Ensure that the firearms policy is consistently enforced. This will help to avoid conflicts down the road when one practitioner allows firearms and another doesn't. Setting a clear policy only goes so far if it's not consistently and fairly enforced.

Overall, the topic of firearms in the community care setting can be problematic if it is not managed and communicated well. However, with the right policies and procedures in place, clear communications, and a consistent approach, most of the issues surrounding firearms in the practice can be mitigated.

CHAPTER 8

Community Care Site Security Operations Models

8.1 Overview

Community care site security operations generally consist of implementing and maintaining layers of security ranging from physical security to training, incident response, and emergency preparedness. Community care site security operations typically fall under one of the following leadership models:

- Practice Manager-Led Security Operations: The practice manager or a similar role is responsible for security operations. In most cases, this responsibility is in addition to myriad other responsibilities from clinical to support operations, facility maintenance coordination, and financial performance. It's not typical for a practice manager to have any formal training or experience in healthcare security to support this responsibility.

- Risk Manager-Led Security Operations: In a multi-site community care organization that is not part of a larger enterprise that includes hospitals, a risk manager, operations manager, or similar role may be tasked with overseeing security operations. Risk managers and operations managers always have other competing priorities, but may have more bandwidth to spend on security operations. However, like practice managers, risk/operations managers usually don't have any healthcare security training or experience to support this responsibility.

- Enterprise-Led Security Operations: When there is a larger enterprise with one or more hospitals as primary/anchor sites, there is typically a professional security department leader who is responsible for the security operations all community care sites. In the case of retail community care settings, the corporate asset protection/loss prevention function typically has responsibility for security operations.

Most community care security operations, regardless of the leadership model in place, don't have resources dedicated to daily security matters. Large medical office buildings or campuses may have permanent on-site security. Also, smaller sites in high-risk locations may have one security officer assigned during operating hours. However, on-site security is rare at most community care sites. Instead, staff at these sites typically rely on local police for emergencies and for non-emergency situations such as threats, stalking/targeting staff, and more.

This chapter focuses on building realistic, effective, and sustainable security operations aligned with the resources and risks within various types of community care organizational models.

8.2   Improved Security Operations Models

There are opportunities for improvements in the current security operations models commonly used by community care organizations. These common security operations models are outlined below along with typical security strategies they employ.

To provide contrast with common strategies employed in the community care setting, summary-level recommendations for improved strategies are also outlined. These improved strategies are designed to offer options to improve the effectiveness of security operations at both individual independent practices and across a healthcare enterprise. In summary, this is an exercise in "how it is" versus "how it could be." The path forward to reach these improved operations models is detailed later in this chapter.

8.2.1   Improved Practice and Risk/Operations Manager - Led Security Operations

Common Leadership Situation: A practice/risk/operations manager or someone in a similar role is tasked with security operations at one or more sites among other competing job priorities. They likely have no formal training or experience in healthcare security and few resources to support this responsibility.

Improved Leadership Situation: A practice/risk/operations manager or someone in a similar role is tasked with security operations at one or more sites among other competing job priorities. Their security-related responsibilities are outlined in their job description, and they are afforded reasonable time and resources to support this responsibility. They have completed appropriate initial and ongoing training to support their security-related responsibilities.

Strategies Employed:

- Routine and Emergency Security Situations:

    - Police Assistance:

        - *Common*: Police are called for emergencies and routine matters such as concerning patient or employee terminations, threats, thefts, etc.

- *Improved*: The practice manager has an established relationship with local police leadership with ongoing proactive meetings each year. Local police are familiar with the site, staff, and their challenges. Police are called for emergencies and routine matters such as concerning patient or employee terminations, threats, etc.

  o Contract Security:

    - *Common*: Contract security staff may be placed on-site when there is a perception of elevated risk based on threats or a recent workplace violence incident. The quality and consistency of security staff can vary widely, expectations of the security staff on site may be unclear on both sides, and the staffing is usually terminated at some point when staff anxiety has subsided.

    - *Improved:* Carefully selected, professional contract security staff are placed on-site when there is a perception of elevated risk based on threats or a recent workplace violence incident. The expectations of the security staff are clearly outlined in writing with the contract security company. The practice manager keeps the company and on-site security staff updated on the situation as it evolves. The decision to continue or terminate security coverage is based on an assessment of the threat situation by a qualified threat assessment and management professional and/or in consultation with law enforcement.

  o Internal Resource(s):

    - *Common*: Staff may be trained to simply summon a certain go-to person(s) in the practice who is perceived as helpful in de-escalating or taking control of escalating situations.

    - *Improved*: Designated members of the leadership and/or staff have received advanced de-escalation and violence training along with emergency management training. Staff are aware of these resources and they can be summoned quickly and reliably.

- Training & Awareness

  o *Common:* There's no workplace violence awareness, security, and/or de-escalation training available for practice staff. Staff may have some training from working at a hospital previously.

  o *Improved*: All staff receive initial and ongoing workplace violence awareness, security, and de-escalation training appropriate for their role and level of risk exposure.

- Policies and Procedures

    - *Common:* There's few (or no) policies and procedures for security and/or violence related emergencies. If policies and procedures are in place, site staff are not trained on them.

    - *Improved:* The following security-related policies and procedures are in place, at minimum, and all staff receive initial and ongoing training on them: workplace violence prevention and mitigation; aggressive/threatening person; lockdown (external threat); active threat/shooter; bomb threat/suspicious package; weapons/firearms; advance planning for problematic patients; patient termination safety measures.

- Physical Security

    - *Common:* Physical security measures, such as card access, cameras, panic alarms, and more may be in place. The practice manager typically leans heavily on vendors/integrators to recommend and maintain these systems. It's common for these measures to be implemented only after an incident(s) prompted concerns about security.

    - *Improved:* Physical security measures are proactively installed based on an initial risk assessment conducted by a qualified independent healthcare security consultant. Ongoing measures are implemented based on evolving risks, industry guidance, standards, and/or best practices.

8.2.2 Improved Enterprise-Led Security Operations

Common Leadership Situation: A security leader is tasked with managing security operations at numerous community care sites spread across a wide geographic area. This responsibility is in addition to numerous other competing job priorities. The security leader has few, if any, dedicated security staff resources focused on or posted at these sites.

Improved Leadership Situation: A community care security manager is focused on security operations at numerous community care sites spread across a wide geographic area. They have a field-based security team that is appropriately sized for the number, geography, and types of community care sites. The field-based team is focused on conducting proactive activities like training and safety planning, supporting non-emergency calls for service, and maintaining close working relationships with site staff.

COMMUNITY CARE SITE SECURITY

Strategies Employed:

- Routine and Emergency Security Situations:
  - Police Assistance:

    - *Common*: Police are called for emergencies and routine matters such as concerning patient or employee terminations, threats, etc.

    - *Improved*: The community care security manager and the practice manager have an established working relationship with local police leadership. The community care security manager is the primary liaison with police leadership. There are proactive meetings with police leadership throughout each year. The community care security team ensures that local police are familiar with the site, their staff, and their challenges. Police are called for emergencies. Routine matters such as concerning patient or employee terminations, threats, etc., are handled by the community care security team as resources permit.

  - Security Staff:

    - *Common*: Despite having a professional security department within the enterprise, contract security staff may be placed at a community care site when there is a perception of elevated risk. The perception of risk may be based on threats or a recent incidence of workplace violence. The quality and consistency of contract security staff can vary widely and expectations of the contract security staff on site may be unclear on both sides.

      If hospital security staff are deployed to a site, it causes a burden on hospital security operations. This is because the enterprise security team is not staffed to support the needs of community care sites. An officer assigned to the site from the hospital likely has no prior relationship with the community care team and it may be their first time at the site.

      Site security staffing is usually terminated at some point when staff anxiety has subsided.

    - *Improved:* Dedicated and specialized community care security staff from the enterprise are deployed to a community care site when needed to address perceived elevated risk. The community care security team, supported at the enterprise level, evaluates the risk and creates a safety plan to prevent or mitigate the threat. The plan is communicated and coordinated with the community care leadership team. The member(s) of the community care security team assigned to the site have good working relationships with staff and are familiar with the site's layout and issues.

The decision to continue or terminate security coverage is based on ongoing assessment of the threat situation by the community care/enterprise security team. The assessment may include consultation with law enforcement, depending on the nature of the threat.

- Internal Resource(s):

  - *Common*: Staff may be trained to simply summon a certain go-to person(s) in the practice who is perceived as helpful in de-escalating or taking control of escalating situations.

  - *Improved*: Designated members of the leadership and/or staff have received advanced de-escalation and violence training from the community care security team along with emergency management training. Staff are aware of these resources, and they can be summoned quickly and reliably. The community care security team keeps the team's preparedness fresh using scenario-based micro-training.

- Training & Awareness

  - *Common:* There's often no workplace violence awareness, security, and/or de-escalation training available for community care site staff. Classes for de-escalation and related topics are held on-site at enterprise hospitals, making it difficult for site staff to attend. Some staff may have training from working at one of the enterprise hospitals previously.

  - *Improved*: All staff receive initial and ongoing workplace violence awareness, security, and de-escalation training appropriate for their role and level of risk exposure. The community care team conducts initial and re-certification training on-site and keeps staff prepared through regular scenario-based micro-training. The training is tailored to the challenges of community care site resources.

- Policies and Procedures

  - *Common:* Policies and procedures for security and/or violence related emergencies are written for enterprise hospitals with different resources and infrastructure than community care sites. If policies and procedures are in place, it's uncommon for site staff to be trained on them.

- o *Improved:* Hospital policies and procedures for security and/or violence related emergencies are customized specifically for the community care operating environment, its resources, and limitations. Staff receive regular and ongoing training on these policies and procedures from the community care security team.

- <u>Physical Security</u>

  - o *Common:* Physical security measures, such as card access, cameras, panic alarms, and more may be in place. The practice manager typically leans heavily on vendors/integrators to recommend and maintain these systems. It's not uncommon for these measures to be implemented only after an incident(s) prompted concerns about security.

  - o *Improved:* The community care security team conducts proactive security risk assessments at each community care site on a regular cadence. The team has implemented minimum physical security standards for all sites in alignment with industry standards. Enhanced security measures beyond this baseline are based on initial and ongoing risk assessments. The team regularly tests panic alarms and ensures other physical security measures are working properly and being used properly by site staff.

8.2.3 Conclusion

The common versus improved strategies outlined in this section are meant to highlight how changing the approach to security operations can result in vastly improved effectiveness. While every site and organization is different, these strategies offer a glimpse into how even small changes can provide safer care environments for staff and patients.

CHAPTER 9

Practice/Operations/Risk Manager-Led Security Operations

9.1 Overview

Practice manager or operations/risk manager-led security operations can be challenging. These managers typically have no formal training or experience in healthcare security. Their security responsibilities are among many other competing responsibilities that range from clinical operations to maintenance issues and human resources functions.

Practice manager-led operations are typical at a standalone, independent community-care site. Operations or risk manager-led security operations are more common in multi-site community care organizations that are not part of a larger healthcare system or organization.

This section outlines a reasonable, realistic approach to security operations led by either role. The approach assumes the leadership challenges outlined here are in place with little to no additional support.

9.2 Security Services

At some point, a practice or operations/risk manager may need to hire a contract security officer(s). A contract security officer is typically hired on a temporary basis in response to an incident that triggered a concern among staff. The types of incidents that can generate fear among staff are usually related to situations such as threats of violence, a recently terminated angry patient, or even an unrelated violent incident at a nearby practice.

The practice or operations/risk manager should identify a good quality, reliable contract security provider before an issue prompts a need for their services. Further, an open, as-needed contract should be established so that procuring a security officer is quick and easy when coverage is needed.

Here are some factors the practice or operations/risk manager should consider when hiring a security officer through a contract security company:

- Low Cost = Low Quality: When it comes to contract security services, you get what you pay for. A lower price means lower quality personnel and services from the contractor. The hourly rate quoted from a security contractor covers everything from officer training to uniforms, benefits, insurance, and a profit margin. A low-price contractor may cut corners to increase profits and place a low-paid security officer at the site with little training or motivation. In the healthcare environment, a high-quality security officer with good de-escalation skills and other relevant training is key. The selection process for contract security services should always be based on quality first and then price.

- Planning and Communication: Planning and communication is key when working with contract security officers. They should be wrapped into the site's team and should have a full understanding of why they are at the site. The officer should also understand what activities are expected of them daily. Bringing in a security officer and then leaving them in the waiting area with no communication and no plan is a recipe for disaster.

- Plainclothes vs. Uniformed: Sometimes a uniformed presence at a site is desired to project authority, a sense of security and to help deter violence. Other times, the presence of a uniformed officer might set someone off or make patients feel uncomfortable visiting your practice. This is especially true if they have negative perceptions about police and security. A plainclothes security officer dressed in normal street clothes or professional attire may be a better option in these situations.

- Armed vs. Unarmed: The decision to hire an armed versus and unarmed security officer should be driven by the situation that prompted hiring the officer. For example, if a patient is making threats to come in and "shoot the place up", the practice may want an armed presence. However, if the situation is related to an angry patient who has an appointment coming up and there's no concerns about weapons, then an unarmed presence may be more suitable. When deciding to hire an armed officer, it is critically important to hire a very high-quality security officer through a reputable and high-quality contract security company. The officer will be carrying a firearm and has the capability of using deadly force to protect themselves and others.

- Multi-tenant Building Security: For practices located within a larger medical office building, it can be tempting to assume that security officer(s) provided by the building management are readily available to help with practice security issues. However, these officers are typically hired for basic security functions and their contract with building management usually limits what they can do. Oftentimes, this means that the officers are limited to an "observe and report" type of role. If they are called by a practice to help with a patient screaming in the waiting room, their response may only be to stand there and act as another witness while calling 911. The only way to understand what services the security officers in a multi-tenant building offer is to ask building management.

Overall, a temporary, quality security officer presence at a practice can enhance the level of safety and security at the site while offering psychological comfort to employees.

9.3 Liaison with Law Enforcement

Interactions with law enforcement shouldn't be limited to emergency situations. Fostering a good working relationship with the local police department can go a long way in improving communications and understanding between practice leadership and the police. Below are key considerations for establishing a good relationship with local law enforcement.

- Meet and Greet: Consider inviting leadership from the local police department to tour the community care site, learn about who it serves, and understand the types of security/violence issues the site staff encounter. When planning a visit by police, ensure that their presence doesn't cause alarm and concern among staff and patients. Provide messaging prior to any visits by the police.

- What to Expect: Find out what to expect when calling the police for assistance. For example, if a staff member calls the police from their cell phone, does it go to a centralized call center that will then transfer it to the local police? What is the average police response time? What is considered a high priority versus a low priority response? And what do the police expect from staff when they show up? Should you meet them outside first? These are all great questions to ask that will help forge better understanding on both sides of the conversation.

- Police Details: Ask local police how to request a detail if one is needed for security related issues in the future. Also ask how much notice is required to fill the detail and the likelihood of filling a detail. Sometimes, competing priorities or a high demand for detail officers can make it difficult for a department to fill all the details requested.

- Protected Health Information and Police: Understand the rules governing what patient information can be shared with law enforcement. There are a lot of misperceptions about what the police can and cannot be told about a patient. Practice leadership and local police leadership should discuss this topic before it becomes a source of conflict in the future.

9.4 Practice Manager Daily Security Operations

Daily security operations for a practice manager should consist of activities that can realistically and consistently fit into their daily routine. A focus on activities with the most return on time invested is key. These activities should be scheduled just like any other important task in the practice manager's schedule to ensure they get done. Here are the core daily security-related activities managers should consider:

- Staff Check-In: Informally check-in with support and clinical staff encountered during the day to identify any security-related concerns they might have such as an upcoming problematic patient visit or a door that won't lock properly. This doesn't mean that every staff member must be interviewed daily, but staff should get used to (and will appreciate) being asked regularly about security issues concerning them. This also allows the manager to anticipate and plan for future issues.

- Site Walk: When walking in and around the community care site, the manager should be alert for the following security-related issues:

    - Staff who may need help with a disruptive or problematic patient.

    - Anxious or upset patients in the waiting area who may need help.

    - Exterior doors propped open.

    - Interior doors leading to staff only areas propped open.

    - Items near doors that might be used to prop them open.

    - Lights out in the parking lot.

    - Persons loitering in the parking lot.

    These are just a few examples of key things that the practice manager can observe while going about their daily duties. However, observing is not enough. The practice manager should take action to address identified concerns.

These daily activities are meant to be realistic given everything else expected of the practice manager. Even though these activities are relatively simple and straightforward, the manager may not be able to accomplish these tasks every day. The key is for the practice manager to make an ongoing effort to have an eye for security and to weave security into everyday activities.

9.4.1 Practice Manager Monthly/Quarterly/Annual Operations

The practice manager should consider conducting the following activities at the corresponding cadence indicated, at minimum:

<u>Monthly Activity</u>

- Test all duress/panic alarms in collaboration with the security systems/alarm vendor. Ensure that any non-working panic alarms are repaired as soon as possible. Non-working alarms should be labeled for staff awareness. Document all activities, including dates of repair.

<u>Quarterly Activity</u>

- Conduct a test of building alarm system devices in collaboration with the security systems/alarm vendor.

<u>Annual Activity</u>

- Conduct a site security and violence risk assessment for the site in collaboration with other site leadership and key stakeholders. After conducting the assessment, create an action plan to address findings and follow-up on the plan through completion.

9.5 Operations/Risk Manager-Led Security Operations

9.5.1 Delegation of Security Operations

Whenever possible, the operations/risk manager should delegate security operations to each practice manager in their site portfolio. This model will help reduce the burden on the operations/risk manager while empowering practice leadership to take charge of their site security.

Accountability for practice managers to accomplish daily/weekly/monthly/annual activities is critically important. If practice managers are not held accountable for their activities, they will likely fall to the wayside of their countless other competing priorities. To achieve accountability and to keep lines of communication open, the operations/risk manager should hold a daily or weekly safety/security video or phone call with all practice leaders to check-in. Further, the operations/risk manager should collect and review all records of regular security operations activities from each practice manager.

9.5.2 Weekly Security Operations

If the operations/risk manager is not able to delegate responsibility for site security operations to each practice manager, they will need to take on these operations themselves. The operations/

risk manager responsible for multiple sites likely doesn't have time to accomplish daily activities at each site. Instead, the manager should plan to complete necessary activities on a weekly basis.

The weekly security operations for the operations/risk manager should consist of activities that can realistically and consistently fit into their routine. A focus on activities with the most return on time invested is key. These activities should be scheduled just like any other important task in the manager's schedule to ensure they get done. Here are the core weekly security-related activities practice managers should consider:

- Practice Manager Check-In: Hold a weekly call with a practice manager from each site to discuss any security issues for the week. These calls should be held on Mondays or Fridays to provide an overview of the coming week and to plan for prevention and/or mitigation strategies. For example, if a site has a patient coming in who has a history of verbal aggression, a plan should be formulated to mitigate the potential risk far in advance of the visit.

- Staff Check-In: Visit each site at least once a week to informally check-in with support and clinical staff to identify any security-related concerns they might have such as an upcoming problematic patient visit or a door that won't lock properly. This doesn't mean that every staff member must be interviewed, but staff should get used to (and will appreciate) being asked regularly about security issues concerning them. This also allows the operations/risk manager to anticipate and plan for future issues.

- Site Walk: When walking in and around each site, the operations/risk manager should do so with an eye for security. Here's some basic things that the manager should look for when walking around:

    o Staff who may need help with a disruptive or problematic patient.

    o Anxious or upset patients in the waiting area who may need help.

    o Exterior doors propped open.

    o Interior doors leading to staff only areas propped open.

    o Items near doors that might be used to prop them open.

    o Lights out in the parking lot.

    o Persons loitering in the parking lot.

These are just a few examples of key things that the operations/risk manager can observe while going about their weekly duties.

However, observing is not enough. The operations/risk manager should take action to address identified concerns and communicate back to practice leadership and staff when issues are resolved. Regular communication with staff about their concerns is helpful, but when staff see that nothing is being done about their concerns, they will lose faith and trust in the leader who is noting concerns but never addressing them. On the other hand, when staff see that their concerns are being taken seriously and being addressed, they will have increased confidence in leadership and will be more likely to report issues in the future.

9.5.3 Monthly/Quarterly/Annual Operations

The operations/risk manager should consider conducting the following activities at the corresponding cadence, at minimum:

<u>Monthly Activity</u>

- Test all duress/panic alarms at each site in collaboration with the security systems/alarm vendor. Ensure that any non-working panic alarms are repaired as soon as possible. Non-working alarms should be labeled for staff awareness. Document all activities, including dates of repair.

<u>Quarterly Activity</u>

- Conduct a test of building alarm system devices at each site in collaboration with the security systems/alarm vendor.

<u>Annual Activity</u>

- The operations/risk manager should conduct a security and violence risk assessment for each site in collaboration with site leadership and key stakeholders annually. This activity should not be delegated to practice managers as it provides an opportunity for the operations/risk manager to audit the risk at each site. After conducting each assessment, create a site portfolio-level action plan to address findings and follow-up on the plan through completion.

CHAPTER 10

Enterprise Security Operations

10.1 Overview

As noted in the previous section, most healthcare enterprises/systems lack a dedicated security leader focused on community care site security. In large healthcare organizations, the number of sites and their spread-out locations can be truly overwhelming for any leader to wrap their arms around. If there is a dedicated leader, chances are that their security staff resources are slim to non-existent.

This chapter covers the process for building an effective and sustainable community care security team from the ground up. For organizations with existing community care security leaders or teams, this section serves as a comparison point and roadmap for improvement.

10.2 Community Care Security Team Strategy

The overarching strategy of community care security operations should be to serve as a resource and partner to community care sites. The typical security strategies employed within hospital security operations may not be a good fit for community care sites. This is because community care sites operate across diverse locations with unique care teams, patient populations, and issues. Therefore, enterprise organizations should consider adopting a community care security strategy using evidence-based practices derived from law enforcement. This strategy can best be described as community-oriented policing in the healthcare setting. The next section describes how each element of community policing can be leveraged to create an effective community care team strategy.

10.2.1 Community Oriented Policing Approach

Community policing is defined by the United Nations (UN) as, "A strategy for encouraging the public to act as partners with the police in preventing and managing crime as well as other aspects of security and order based on the needs of the community" (USG DPKO, USG DFS, 2018). In the community care setting, the "community" consists of the staff, patients, contractors, and visitors at each community care site. The "police" for the community consists of the community care security team, who may or may not have law enforcement powers.

The UN has created four cornerstones of community-oriented policing that the community care security team can adopt as part of their approach:

1. "Consulting with communities- regular solicitation of input from communities about crime, disorder, and activities that generate fear;
2. Responding to communities -willingness and ability to respond to the security needs of individuals and groups in communities and to give priority to these needs;
3. Mobilizing communities - helping the community organize itself in controlling crime; and
4. Solving recurring problems - police and communities working preventively to change conditions that lead to crime rather than responding over and over again to individual incidents" (USG DPKO, USG DFS, 2018).

10.2.2 Community-Oriented Policing Effectiveness

The effectiveness of community policing has been studied extensively over the past several decades. Studies have indicated that the positive effects of community-oriented policing include, but are not limited to, reduction in fear of crime, increased trust of the police and reporting of crimes, and satisfaction with police.

For example, a meta-analysis of fifty community policing studies by Zhao et. al. (2006) found that, in most of the studies (31), there was a reduction in fear of crime among citizens. However, eighteen of the studies indicated no change in fear of crime and one study found an increase in fear of crime (Zhao et al., 2006). These findings around decreases in fear of crime are consistent with research conducted by Roh & Oliver in 2005.

Another meta-analysis conducted by Gill et al. in 2014 did not find the same positive impacts on fear of crime as Zhao et al. (2006), but interestingly found that community-oriented policing increased trust in the police and satisfaction with services rendered by law enforcement. These positive effects resulted in an increased likelihood for people to report crimes and other issues to police (Gill et al., 2014).

While these studies were focused on community-oriented policing in a public setting, they point to the potential effectiveness of leveraging this approach to reduce fear of crime and improving relationships between community care site staff and the community care security team.

10.2.3 Adapting Community-Oriented Policing for Community Care Security

Community-oriented policing should be adopted by community care security team as part of the overall operational strategy. Here's how the four cornerstones of community-oriented policing outlined by the UN can be leveraged as part of this strategy:

1. Consulting with site communities:

    a. The community care security team should informally connect with site staff and leadership when on-site and ask them what security, crime, or other concerns they have both on-site and in the community.

    b. When possible, community care security team members should attend site staff meetings, leadership meetings, and/or site safety team meetings to identify concerns.

2. Responding to site communities:

    a. To build and maintain trust with community care sites, the community care security team must be responsive when site staff bring issues to their attention. This is especially true because the community care security team is likely the primary or only connection the site has to the enterprise security department. The community care security team members should regularly provide updates to site staff on how they are responding to concerns.

    b. Issues that are community-related require the community care security team to leverage their relationships with local police to help address concerns. Similar to the community care security team being the primary connection for the site to enterprise security, they are most likely the primary connection to the local police.

3. Mobilizing site communities:

    a. An important part of the community care security team role is to ensure that staff are empowered to respond to security-related situations through initial and ongoing training. Site staff must understand the violence safety gap at their site and how to stay safe from the start of a workplace violence incident until police arrive.

    b. At larger community care sites, the community care security team may organize and train an internal crisis response team to help respond to security and violence related emergencies.

4. Solving recurring problems:

    a. Ultimately, site communities and community care security teams need to work together to develop strategies and tactics to address ongoing issues. Some of these issues will be common across multiple sites.

Leveraging the four cornerstones of community-oriented policing can provide an effective pathway to building and fostering relationships with community care site communities. These relationships can support ongoing security and violence prevention/mitigation efforts while empowering site staff.

CHAPTER 11

Establishing the Community Care Security Team

11.1 Leadership

The community care security team needs a security leader focused on overseeing its operations. The size of the site portfolio should drive the amount of focused time needed to run community care security operations. For example, a single community hospital with only fifteen sites spread across a small geographic area, the leader may need to focus 20% or less of their time on leading security operations. In contrast, a large enterprise with hundreds of sites spread across a wide geography may require a leader dedicated 100% to oversight of community care security operations.

Further, the leader's title should be aligned with the size of the program, the size of the enterprise, and their level of autonomy and responsibility. A smaller site portfolio with minimal leadership autonomy and responsibility may warrant a manager-level professional. On the other hand, a larger site portfolio in a large enterprise with high leadership autonomy and responsibility may warrant a director-level professional. Regardless of the title, the leader should have direct line reporting to the senior leader of the enterprise security operation or another appropriate high-level security leader.

The community care security team leader should regularly meet and communicate with the senior organizational leader responsible for community care site operations and should attend relevant community care site meetings. The idea here is to weave the community care security team into site and clinical operations. Greater collaboration with community care operations means a more effective security team.

11.2 Staffing

Small community care portfolios are typically served using existing security team members. In smaller operations, the ability to visit sites with regular frequency can be challenging given limited resources. It's also unlikely that specialized community care security team roles would be utilized for this work.

However, larger scale community care portfolios require dedicated security staff focused on security operations across these sites. The number of staff needed should be based on a combination of the following factors:

Site Factors:

- Total number of sites
- Geographic diversity of locations, (i.e., distance between sites)
- Services offered at each site (e.g.- behavioral health, surgical, urgent care)
- Hours of operation at each site
- Size of individual sites
- Security incident data
- Crime risk at each site

Security Program Factors:

- Desired level of service to sites*

- Frequency of security site visits desired (i.e., daily, weekly, monthly, etc.)

    o Frequency of site visits will also drive the level of engagement with site staff and leadership.

- Current state of physical security at sites (i.e., well-established, inconsistent, non-existent, etc.).

- Current state of operational security, such as training, preparedness, etc. (i.e., well-established, inconsistent, non-existent, etc.).

- Budgetary constraints

*Note that most community care security teams do not have the capability to reliably replace police as first responders to emergencies.

There's no mathematical formula that incorporates these factors to spit out the right number of staff needed. However, through careful consideration of each factor, it should be possible to identify the minimum number of staff to get the program off the ground initially. The data collected, feedback from site leadership, and other information gathered in this step will help to lobby for budgetary resources to build the program.

CHAPTER 12

The Community Care Security Officer (CCSO)

12.1 Overview

The Community Care Security Officer (CCSO), a term created for this manual, is a specialized position that is designed to meet the needs of community care sites - particularly in larger enterprises. The CCSO should be able to operate in the field with minimal supervision and high autonomy. They should have a bias for action and outstanding communication and problem-solving skills. To be successful, the CCSO should have the training, support, and resources needed to execute their mission.

Given the expectations of the CCSO role, it should be a step above a security officer within the hierarchy of the department with a salary to match the level of responsibility and autonomy of the position. The role should be considered prestigious and a step up the career ladder towards future leadership positions. Depending on the organization, this position may be best aligned with a Lead Officer role, which sits between an officer and a supervisor position. In smaller organizations, one or more officers can be cross trained to assume the responsibilities of the CCSO, but may not be assigned this role on a permanent and dedicated basis.

12.2 Selection

Community Care Security Officers (CCSOs) should be selected from applicants within the existing security team whenever possible. It's important that candidates have been with the security team long enough for department leadership to assess their capabilities and future potential. Further, all candidates should be required to apply for and interview for the position rather than being selected or "volun-told". CCSOs must be invested and committed to the role, which requires that they take the first step and apply for the position. The ideal CCSO candidate should have the following minimum qualities and skills:

- Trustworthy and capable of operating in the field with minimal supervision.
- Proactive with a bias for action.

- Self-starter with the ability to identify and solve security and non-security issues.
- Good judgement in normal and high-stress situations.
- Eager to learn and understand community care site operations.
- Excellent communication and relationship building skills.
- Above average writing ability to produce reports.
- Good time management and ability to handle competing priorities.
- Ability to train others after completion of a train-the-trainer course.

12.3 Training

The CCSO should receive training beyond what is typical for a security officer role within the department. Additional training considerations include, but are not limited to:

- International Association for Healthcare Security and Safety (IAHSS):
  - Basic Officer Certification
  - Advanced Officer Certification

- Security risk assessment training
- Community-oriented policing basics
- Train-the-trainer certification in the preferred de-escalation program

Ultimately, the training required of CCSOs should match the expectations for their role and the goals of the community care site security program.

12.4 CCSO Operations

12.4.1 Field-Based Team

Community Care Security Officers (CCSOs) should be based in the field. They will need to either use their own vehicle or an organization-provided vehicle to visit their assigned sites. Consider having CCSOs based at a high/elevated risk community care site rather than out of a main hospital site. This will provide more problematic sites with a regular presence and allow the CCSO to become embedded within the site's team.

12.4.2 Daily Operations

Daily operations and activities of the security team should primarily be proactive. Below is an outline of typical daily activities that should be expected of a CCSO:

- Conduct Training:
  - Scenario-based micro-training
- Relationship Building:
  - Practice manager, leadership, staff
  - Local police leadership
- Information Gathering:
  - Interact with site staff to boost perceptions about security support and presence. Seek to identify concerns among staff.
  - Identify upcoming/ongoing issues with patients, staff, and others.
  - Identify surrounding community issues that impact the site such as crime, parking, and neighborhood conflicts.
- Problem identification/resolution
  - Identify and address security issues.
  - Ask about and assist site staff with addressing non-security issues (facilities, business, or operational) where appropriate.
  - Place and track work orders for security and/or facility-related issues.
- Site Patrol:
  - Outer/exterior perimeter
  - Inner/interior perimeter
  - Treatment areas
  - Electronic security systems functionality
  - Security and/or safety issue identification

The daily, weekly, and monthly activities of CCSOs should be outlined in a comprehensive post order. Further, a site checklist should be employed to ensure that team members complete all required activities at each site. All activities should also be consistently documented in the department's electronic security log.

12.4.3 Monthly/Quarterly/Annual Operations

The following activities and cadence should be considered, at minimum:

Monthly Activities

- Test all duress/panic alarms. Submit work orders for and properly label non-working devices. Document all activities, including dates of repair.
- Conduct scheduled initial or refresher de-escalation training.
- Attend community care site security team meetings and share information, strategies, successes, and issues.

Quarterly Activities

- Submit a high-level report outlining key activities (training, testing, problem identification and resolution) completed during the quarter within the assigned area to the community care security team leader.
- Conduct a test of building alarm system devices.

Annual Activities

- Conduct a comprehensive site security and violence risk assessment for all locations within assigned area. These site risk assessments should be scheduled at the beginning of each year to ensure that they can all be completed during the year and to prevent a bottleneck of risk assessments at the end of each year.
- Submit a high-level report for all activities completed within the assigned area during the year using the quarterly activity reports.

12.4.4 Special Operations - Security Details

CCSOs may need to perform security details at sites when there is a potential issue, such as a patient conflict or high-risk employee termination. It's critical that officers encourage site staff to notify them as far in advance as possible when details are needed. This will help ensure that coverage can be arranged by the officer or another team member.

Prior to any detail where there is a concern for violence, the team member should perform a threat assessment in collaboration with the community care site leadership, human resources (for employee matters), the security team leader, and the enterprise security team. The threat assessment should also be used to determine the number of security staff needed on-site and whether an armed officer or police detail is needed.

CCSOs should always notify the community care security team leader and their security operations center about any details and the approximate start and end time for officer safety and accountability.

12.5 Essential CCSO Equipment

12.5.1 Field Communications

Maintaining regular communications in the field is essential for the safety and accountability of CCSOs. CCSOs may need to be issued a smartphone by the organization to provide community care sites with a non-personal phone number to reach them during business hours. Further, two-way radios can facilitate regular and emergency communications with the organization's security operations center and other CCSOs. However, in a wide geographic area, traditional two-way radios will likely fail to operate reliably unless the organization has a very robust regional radio repeater network.

Updated two-way radio technology can now operate on cellular networks, providing reliable radio communications in areas with reliable cellular network coverage. This technology can allow radios to operate wherever a cell phone would work- enabling CCSOs to speak with one another and the primary security operations center (SOC) from virtually anywhere. Some technology, like the Motorola WAVE PTX, can also allow the SOC to track the real time location of CCSOs and offer a panic alarm feature.

Lastly, the CCSO should have an encrypted laptop with virtual private network (VPN) access assigned to them so that they can document incidents and activities in the field, log activities, submit work orders, etc.

CHAPTER 13

Community Care Site Intelligence Operations

13.1 Overview

Intelligence operations for community care sites includes sourcing, collecting, analyzing, and distributing information that is useful to the safety and security of these sites. Since sites are often spread across a wide geographic area, it's important to have a consistent feed of information regarding potential issues and hazards that could impact site operations. Ideally, the sourcing and collection of information in this case is automated through a specialized intelligence platform. However, it's not enough to simply collect this information- it must be analyzed and leveraged to enhance site safety, security, and business continuity.

13.2 Intelligence Collection Technology

If the enterprise has a security operations center, the community care sites should be incorporated into the center. Ideally, the center should monitor intelligence feeds regarding incidents that may impact the safety, security, and/or operations of community care sites. Issues that could impact community care sites that should be monitored in real-time at the SOC include, but are not limited to:

- External serious violent crime in progress
- Civil unrest/protest
- Major fire or HAZMAT situation nearby
- Road closures
- Severe weather
- Utility outages

There are several different cloud-based solutions providers that offer such intelligence feeds for multiple locations. These solutions can typically be configured to alert SOC operators to issues of concern that can be relayed to the security team and practice leadership. Examples of these Software as a Service (SaaS) products include, but are not limited to: AlertMedia, Dataminr, Factal, and Hozint.

13.3 Intelligence Alerting

SOC personnel should have a means to communicate urgent issues directly, quickly, and effectively to practice leadership and/or staff via a notification system and direct phone contact. Calling the practice main number and going through a phone tree followed by hold time is not a viable notification strategy. An existing mass notification system can be used to facilitate such alerts by geofencing the alert distribution to locations impacted only. Depending on the type of system in place, desktop alerts could also immediately notify staff of life-threatening situations.

CCSOs should also receive any alerts sent by the SOC to their assigned sites and ideally should receive real-time alerts directly from the chosen SaaS intelligence platform.

13.4 Field Intelligence

CCSOs should seek to collect intelligence in the field from local police, fire, government, and other sources. They should also follow up on intelligence that could impact sites in the future, such as road closures, severe weather, and planned demonstrations.

The CCSO should take the initial lead in verifying any intelligence information received before communicating it. Once verified, identified issues should be communicated to community care site leadership, the community care security leader, the SOC, and other leadership as appropriate. Depending on the nature of the issue, the CCSO should help facilitate any advance planning for the incident in collaboration with key stakeholders.

FINAL THOUGHTS

Whether you're a practice manager at an independent doctor's office, a security leader in a large healthcare organization, or anyone in between, I hope this manual has provided you with the guidance and motivation you need to build an effective, sustainable community care security program.

Through reading this manual, you've learned about everything from calculating the violence safety gap to planning for problematic patients, and more. Each chapter has outlined cost effective, actionable strategies and tactics – many of which you can start implementing right away. You've even been equipped with a step-by-step process to evaluate everything from workplace violence risk at each site to proper lighting in the parking lot.

What I'm trying to say is that I hope that I accomplished my mission of empowering you and your team to build a more secure community care environment while preventing and mitigating the persistent threat of violence.

Now the question is how are you going to apply the knowledge and insights from this manual? What will you start doing today to improve your security measures and operations? Keep the momentum you have right now to start making a difference today. Make a plan, get leadership support, and move the needle forward towards a better future for your colleagues and patients.

Thank you for everything you are doing to improve the security of community care sites. I am truly grateful for your efforts, whether they are small or large. Every little bit helps, so don't stop trying to improve every day.

With Gratitude,

David Corbin

David P. Corbin, CPP, CPHA
Healthcare Violence & Security Consultant, Author

How to Reach David Corbin

Please don't hesitate to reach out to me if I can be of any assistance to you or your healthcare organization. I truly enjoy helping others.

Here's how you can connect with me…

Learn more: www.DavidPCorbin.com
Join my professional community: linkedin.com/in/davecorbincpp/
Email me: Dave@DavidPCorbin.com

You can reach out to me for:

- Security Risk Assessment – I will help you identify security and violence risks within your organization and recommend cost-effective, sustainable prevention and mitigation solutions.

- Workplace Violence Prevention & Mitigation – I will assess your current workplace violence risks, help you develop effective prevention and mitigation strategies and tactics, and build a compliant, effective program.

- Training, Education & Speaking Opportunities – I speak and train teams on healthcare violence and security for audiences including clinical, support, and security teams. I leverage extensive experience teaching at the university level and creating professional development programs for organizations large and small to build engaging, effective training.

- Security Department Enhancement – I will help you enhance your security department's effectiveness, operations, training, use-of-force protocols, violence prevention efforts, and more. I also offer security leadership coaching for new and existing leaders.

- Virtual/Fractional Security Leadership – I offer the benefits of an experienced healthcare security leader when you don't have the budget or need for a full-time position.

These are examples of the most popular services I offer. If you don't see what you're looking for, please reach out to discuss how I can help you and your organization.

ABOUT THE AUTHOR

David Corbin is a healthcare violence and security consultant. He is the author of the *Patient Violence Prevention and Mitigation Field Manual*, a top-rated resource used by healthcare leaders around the globe.

David and his healthcare security strategies have been featured in Chief Healthcare Executive, OBR Oncology, Health Facilities Management, Campus Safety, The Boston Globe and the IAHSS Journal of Healthcare Protection Management.

He has honed his specialization in healthcare violence prevention and security over more than two decades. Using creativity and innovation, he has built highly effective security operations in several challenging environments from the ground up. David previously served as the Director of Police, Security and Parking at Brigham and Women's Hospital/Brigham Health, where he built a comprehensive violence prevention and mitigation program and initiated the complete transformation of the 125-person Police & Security Department. As an Adjunct Professor at the Northeastern University School of Criminology and Criminal Justice, David developed and taught security management courses.

Under David's leadership, the Police & Security Department at Faulkner Hospital won the prestigious Lindberg Bell Award in 2011 for establishing and maintaining an outstanding security program. He is also the 2016 recipient of the IAHSS Philip A. Gaffney Faculty Chair Award for his writings and works toward the furtherance of professionalism in the healthcare security field.

David holds credentials as a Certified Protection Professional (CPP), Certified Healthcare Protection Administrator (CHPA), and Certified Crime Prevention Through Environmental Design (CPTED) Specialist. He is a graduate of both the Gavin de Becker & Associates Advanced Threat Assessment and Management Academy and the Wharton/ASIS Security Executive Program. David holds a master's degree in criminal justice from Northeastern University in Boston, MA and a bachelor's degree in criminal justice from Roger Williams University in Bristol, RI.

He consults and advocates for healthcare security and violence prevention/mitigation internationally.